ESPECIALLY FOR WOMEN

Strength Training
Exercise
Diet
Nutrition

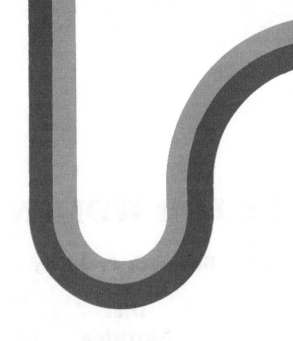

ESPECIALLY

FOR WOMEN

Ellington Darden, Ph.D.

Leisure Press
P.O. Box 3
West Point, N.Y. 10996

A publication of Leisure Press.
P.O. Box 3, West Point, N.Y. 10996
Copyright © 1977 by Ellington Darden
All rights reserved. Printed in the U.S.A.

Library of Congress Catalog Card No. 76-62812

ISBN 0-918438-00-4

Cover Photographs by Ken Neely and Inge Cook
Graphics by Lee Fulford

Contents

Preface

While finshing my post-doctoral study at Florida State University in 1973, I appeared on the Mike Douglas television show. During the interview, I was asked what I planned to do after my study was completed.

"Dispel old myths that surround exercise and nutrition," I replied.

I am interested in dispelling the myths that surround exercise and nutrition because I have made so many mistakes in both. As a teenage athlete I believed all the "old wives' tales" or, more correctly, "old men's locker room tales." I exercised, in the wrong fashion, to get stronger. I also wore a rubber sweat belt around my waist to lose fat there. I swallowed vitamin pills for super health and drank wheat germ oil for stamina. I had a whole list of "do's" and "don't's" that was guaranteed to make me a champion.

After ten years of going through every exercise gimmick and food fad imaginable, I changed my views. This was largely due to the influence of two men, Dr. Harold E. Schendel and Arthur A. Jones. Dr. Schendel was my professor in the Food and Nutrition Department at Florida State University. Arthur Jones is the President of the Nautilus Sports/Medical Industries. Both these men advocate going back to the basic chemistry and physics of the human body for solutions to physical problems.

Since I have believed in the fads as well as the facts of exercise and nutrition, I am in a position to choose between them. Facts, logical facts, based on chemical and physical laws are the basis of my present beliefs concerning bodily health and strength.

But what about you? Are you wasting money on worthless, or even dangerous, exercise and diet fads?

Women are generally more body conscious than men. They are also more food and health conscious. Therefore, many of my articles in both scientific journals and popular magazines have been directed toward women. I have supervised the training of several hundred women at Florida State University and the Athletic Center of Atlanta, Georgia. I have also spoken to many women's groups that were interested in physical fitness and nutrition. All of them expressed a desire for factual printed material that was readily available.

Such material is scarce. Most of that which has been published is in obscure journals that are difficult to locate in university libraries. Many women say they have been unable to find my articles when they needed them.

Especially For Women, therefore, is a compilation of non-technical, easy-to-understand articles about exercise and nutrition. Some of the material has been previously published. Whether previously published or specially written for this book, each selection is designed to stand by itself as a separate article.

This book covers a wide range of topics. Part A begins with a series of articles on strength training specially designed for women. When all factors are considered, women may actually have more to gain from strength training than men.

The articles in Part B concern fitness-related topics. Such activities as jogging, swimming, and bicycling are discussed. Special exercises for pregnant women are explained.

The final section, Part C, deals with diet and nutrition. Some of the subjects treated are how to evaluate nutritional status, how to lose body fat, and how to select and store fresh fruits and vegetables for maximum nutrition.

Especially For Women offers something for all women from pre-teens to grandmas—from athletes to loungers—from beauty queens to plain Janes. The conclusions in this book are based largely on physical and chemical facts. It is designed to produce results.

PART
A
STRENGTH TRAINING

INTRODUCTION TO STRENGTH TRAINING

The first article, "You're Stronger Than You Think!" takes a hard look at the controversial subject of strength training for women. Six highly esteemed "old wives' tales" are put to rest and the basic rules of building strength are discussed. In addition, specific exercises for various sports are listed.

"Dimples, Pockmarks, and Ripples," those unsightly formations that many women have on their buttocks and how to prevent or eliminate them, are the areas for discussion in the next article. The recommended exercises are also very important to female athletes, since the buttocks are the strongest muscles of the body and are used in all sports that require running and jumping.

Article three is concerned with the body part that 95% of the women in the United States are dissatisfied with: the bustline. If exercise can help chest development, then the movements in this program will do it.

"Three Steps to a Slim, Trim Waistline" is the title of the next article. Proper exercise can do just so much for your waist. Posture and diet are of equal importance. You will learn why in the fourth selection.

Tennis may be the most popular sport of all for women. However, many women are not strong enough to obtain a moderate level of success in tennis. The ones who are would do even better if their muscles were stronger. Article five gives a step by step account of building strength for tennis.

The next article covers one of the most important, yet most vulnerable part of the female anatomy: the knees. What can you do to protect and prevent injury to your knees? You will find the answer in six.

What about strength for older women? Do not despair. Article seven was written specially for the over fifty age group.

"Something for Men," article eight, answers frequently asked questions that men have about strength training, muscles, fat, and exercise in general. Perhaps you have men friends who would find these facts interesting.

You're
Stronger
Than You
Think

1

YOU'RE STRONGER THAN YOU THINK

Give me 15 minutes of your day and I'll take sleeping muscles already present in your body and build them up.

---Charles Atlas

If Charles Atlas were alive and flexing the last place he would run an ad would be in a book for women. The mistake would be a natural one---but a mistake, nevertheless.

Research shows that a body-building program of progressive resistance can offer as much to women as the familiar ninety-seven pound weakling of the comic book ads did for men. The gains would be in strength, not in bulging muscles.

That's right! It's possible to have the strength of Charles Atlas without looking like him.

Strength is a major component of all physical activities, because muscles, by contracting and relaxing, move our bodies. The stronger your muscles are, the more efficiently you move; and it doesn't matter if you are a teenager, an expectant mother, a housewife or a grandma. If you strengthen your muscles, you'll be a better teenager, mother, housewife, or grandma. All women athletes should take notice: if you increase the strength of the muscles directly involved in your sport, you'll be a better athlete.

Before getting to the basic principles of building strength, let's clear the ground of certain exercise myths or "old wives' tales."

OLD WIVES' TALES

Large Muscles

Most women believe that if they participate in heavy exercise, they'll develop large, unfeminine muscles. The truth is that it's practically impossible for a woman to develop large muscles.

It's no accident that men develop larger, more defined muscle mass. This is the result of the male hormone testosterone upon the growth mechanism of the male's body.

Before puberty, there's little difference between the muscular size and strength of boys and girls. With the onset of puberty, testosterone from the boy's testes and estrogen from a girl's ovaries enter the bloodstream and influence muscular growth.

There are a small percentage of women who have large muscles, particularly in their legs. These muscles are either inherited or are the result of an abnormally high amount of testosterone in the system.

The adrenal glands and the sex glands within both men and women secrete a small amount of the nondominant hormone. As a result, there are a few women who have inherited large muscles and at the same time have a large amount of testosterone in their systems.

These women do have the potential to develop muscles. There are also men who have an extra amount of estrogen in their systems. This tends to give them a feminine appearance.

Generally speaking, 99% of American women could not develop large muscles if their lives depended upon it. But, heavy exercise is worthwhile because it strengthens and conditions your muscles. This, in turn, will make you a better athlete.

The idea that women are inferior to men in muscular strength is somewhat related to these Old Wives' Tales.

Strength: Women versus Men

This topic was recently studied by Dr. C. Harmon Brown and Dr. Jack H. Wilmore of the University of California at Davis. They placed forty-seven college aged women and twenty-six college aged men, all of whom were untrained, on a ten-week weight training program.

After the program was over, both groups had made substantial gains in strength. In terms of actual weight lifted, the upper body strength of men was 50% higher than that of the women. The lower body strength was 25% higher for men. However, when they figured leg strength relative to lean body weight (total of weight minus the weight of fat), the women rated 5.8% stronger than the men.

In the final analysis, Dr. Wilmore concludes: " . . . if you look at strength in terms of size of the individual-- minus fat-- you find that the strength potential is theoretically similar for men and women."

Let us move on to the myth that strong muscles make you less flexible or " muscle bound."

Lack of Flexibility

Flexibility is related to your ability to stretch and contract your muscles throughout a full range of movement. Over 434 skeletal muscles are responsible for your overall movement potential.

Muscles were tailor-made to be used. The "use it or lose it" maxim applies nowhere as cogently as here. You can actually lose some of the range of motion of a particular muscle if it is not used throughout its full stretching and contracting process. In other words, you become "muscle bound" from using your muscles *too little*, not too much. This can easily be observed in the inflexible walk or shuffle that most elderly people develop.

Proper strength-training programs apply resistance to your muscles as they are stretched and contracted. Muscles that have been conditioned in this manner are not only strong but flexible. This was proven in 1975 by Dr. Jim Peterson of the United States Military Academy in testing Cadets before and after a six-week strength-training program.

As an added attraction, when you increase the strength of a muscle, you also increase the power to weight ratio. This means that your speed of movement will be improved. In other words, you'll be faster.

Speed of movement also relates to the amount of fat that you have in your body. Fat between muscle fibers acts as a friction brake and can actually impede the normal, relatively frictionless contraction of lean muscle fibers. Therefore, it is important to understand the difference between muscle and fat.

Composition of Muscle and Fat

	water	lipids	proteins
MUSCLE	70%	7%	22%
FAT	22%	72%	6%

A pound of fat has 3,500 calories while a pound of muscle contains only 600 calories. Most of muscle is water, but fatty tissue is composed mainly of fat. The density of muscle is much greater than that of fat.

A common misconception among athletes is that muscles are made of protein, and to get stronger muscles you must eat massive amounts of proteins. This is simply not true! Seventy percent of muscle is water, not protein.

Athletes with high levels of muscular strength who suddenly quit training get significant reductions (atrophy) in muscle mass as well as reductions in overall calorie requirements. Thus, the athlete who stops training should reduce her caloric intake accordingly. What usually occurs if this is not done is a slow increase in the percentage of body fat and a decrease in the percentage of muscle mass, even though her bodyweight may remain relatively stable.

Fat Distribution

As women get older, they tend to deposit fat around the hips and thighs, while men are likely to deposit it in the abdomen and as a roll around the sides.

While the energy balance (intake vs. output) determines the amount of fat present, other factors determine the way it is distributed over the body. The most important factor is inheritance. Just as different races and different families have characteristic heights, coloring, and nose shapes, they also have characteristic patterns of fat distribution.

Hormones also influence the distribution of body fat. Androgens and estrogens are largely responsible for the way men and women deposit fat. The breasts, for example, are mostly fat, not glandular tissue as many people imagine; and estrogens are particularly responsible for this fat deposition.

Exercise and Fat Reduction

Most people believe that concentrated exercise for a particular body part that is laden with fat will be effective in removing fat (spot reduction). Although exercise does play a part in the reduction of body fat (along with proper diet), fat is mobilized out of multiple fat cells all over the body. Thus, spot reducing is impossible.

In order to reduce your percentage of body fat, you have to force your body to burn its own fat as a source of energy. Consuming 1,000 less calories a day than is required for your maintenance level, will require your body to burn several pounds of fat a week as a source of energy. But, even then, fat will come from all over your body, not just one spot.

Remember, the areas and the order in which you store fat have been genetically determined. Try as you may, you cannot change it. This does not mean that proper exercise will not benefit you. Proper exercise will strengthen your muscles, and the fat and skin that surround these muscles will become tighter and firmer. In short, you'll be more physically attractive.

STRENGTH BUILDING PRINCIPLES

In 1945 scientific experimentation and clinical application by Dr. Thomas Delorme of Harvard Medical School proved that the best way to build strength was through a program of progressive resistance exercise. This conclusion has been reconfirmed many times in the last thirty years. An exercise is progressive only if it involves constantly increasing workloads each training session. Such exercise can be performed by using a variety of equipment such as barbells, dumbbells, or weight machines. Good results can be obtained from almost any equipment if several training principles are understood.

Intensity

The building of strength is related to the intensity of exercise: the higher the intensity, the better the muscles are stimulated. High-intensity exercise is best defined as the repetitive performance of a resistance movement that is carried to the point of momentary muscular failure. Practical experience shows that at least eight repetitions should be performed and not more than twelve. When you can perform twelve repetitions in good form, that is a signal to increase the resistance by approximately 5% in that exercise at the time of the next workout. But the real key to technique is pushing yourself, or being pushed by someone else, in an all-out effort. Consider a set completed when it is momentarily impossible to perform another repetition in good form.

Form or Style

Good form or style is very important if maximum benefit is to be obtained from strength training. Proper form includes: (1) the speed of movement, (2) the range of movement, (3) beginning the movement from a pre-stretched position.

The speed of movement must not be too fast or too slow. The resistance should be moved in a smooth fashion and briefly stopped in the position of full muscular contraction. Jerking movements should be avoided. Research by Dr. Paavo Komi of Finland has shown that for building strength, lowering the resistance (eccentric or negative contraction) is far more important than raising the resistance. A good rule of thumb is: if it takes two seconds to lift a weight, then it should take four seconds or twice as long to lower that weight. It should take at least one minute to complete a set of ten repetitions using correct form.

The range of movement must be as great as possible. In order to contract, a muscle must produce movement. In order to contract fully, a muscle must produce a full range of possible movement. If the movement resulting from the muscular contraction is less than the full range the entire length of the muscle is not involved in the work. In addition, prevention of injury is most likely when the muscles have been strengthened in every position over a full range of possible movement.

The movement must start from a pre-stretched position. Pre-stretching is involved when a relaxed muscle is pulled into a position of increased tension prior to the start of contraction. Pre-stretching properly applied enables you to handle heavier weights and thus bring into action a greater percentage of muscle mass during each repetition. For example, the weight should be lowered from the contracted position in a controlled manner until the bar (resistance arm) is about one inch from a position of full stretch. At that point, there should be a very quick "twitch" or "thrust." Immediately following this quick "twitch," the movement should be slowed down in a controlled manner The only rapid movement of the bar or resistance arm should be during the last portion of the lowering (negative) part of the repetition and the first portion of the raising (positive) part of the repetition. The remaining part of each repetition should be smoothly performed.

Duration and Frequency

If the exercise is done using the high-intensity principle, with special emphasis on good form, the workouts themselves must be brief. A workout should consist of no more than twelve exercises (four to six for the lower body and six to eight for the upper body). Perform only one set of each exercise and take no longer than thirty minutes to complete the entire routine.

Phenomenal strength gains from such brief training have been repeatedly demonstrated in the Exercise Physiology laboratory at Colorado State University by Dr. Eliot Plese.

Time between workouts is also important. Best results occur when there are at least forty-eight hours between workouts and not more than ninety-six hours. The only exception to this principle would be during the early stages of rehabilitation where the intensity of work is so low that training is possible on a daily basis. This means if you are a beginning trainee, you should train every other day. Advanced trainees, because they handle much heavier resistance with more intensity, must train even less---only two times a week.

Remember, brief workouts two or three times a week are best for building strength.

Sequence

Begin all workouts with the largest muscle group and proceed down to the smallest. You may wonder why. Strength expert Arthur Jones says that it is sometimes impossible to reach the required condition of momentary muscular exhaustion while working a large muscle group if the system has been previously exhausted by exercises for other smaller muscles. Therefore it is important to work the largest muscles first while the system is still capable of working to the required degree.

With this in mind, the order of exercise should be: hips, legs, back, shoulders, chest, and arms.

Recommended Exercises

The four basic principles of building strength can be used with barbells, dumbbells, and various weight machines. I have trained small groups of women with satisfactory results from both barbell exercises and weight-machines exercises (Universal Gym machines and Nautilus machines). However, superior strength gains occured when women were trained on the Nautilus machines.

Nautilus machines are especially good for women because they eliminate the weak points in barbell-related exercises. Barbell exercises, for example, for the upper body must be performed by gripping the bar; since women's hands and arms are much weaker than their torso muscles, the weaker muscles tire before the stronger muscles can be completely worked. This is overcome in the Nautilus machines because the resistance is directly applied to the appropriate part of the body.

Nautilus machines also provide rotary movement, variable resistance, balance resistance, and muscular stretching-----all the requirements for full-range exercise. As a result, maximum increases in strength can be produced in much less training time than previously thought possible.

A basic strength-training program utilizing Nautilus machines or conventional equipment would look something like the following chart. First, though, a word of caution, be sure to allow at least one week's time for a gradual break-in process to take place. Use light resistance in all movements and practice correct form. After a week or so, you may then progress in high-intensity fashion. These are the exercises you will need:

NAUTILUS MACHINES	CONVENTIONAL EQUIPMENT
1. Hip and Back	1. Squat (barbell)
2. Leg Extension	2. Pullover (barbell plate)
3. Leg Press	3. Stiff-legged deadlift (barbell)
4. Leg Curl	4. Press (barbell)
5. Pullover	5. Curl (barbell)
6. Torso-Arm	6. Bench press (barbell)
7. Double Shoulder	7. Shoulder shrug (barbell)
a. Lateral raise	
b. Overhead press	
8. Neck and Shoulder	8. Sit-up (accentuate lowering)
9. Double Chest	9. Chin-up (horizontal bar, accentuate lowering)
a. Arm cross	
b. Decline press	10. Dip (parallel bars, accentuate lowering

In the last fifty years Charles Atlas ads convinced millions of men to believe:"You're Stronger Than You Think!" Hopefully, you now believe that you are stronger than you think----or at least your potential for strength is greater than you previously thought.

Yes, it is possible to have the strength of Charles Atlas without looking like him. Just apply the four principles of building strength to your training programs and watch what happens to your "sleeping muscles."

At least you will be prepared next time you are on the beach and some bully kicks sand in your face!

1. HIP AND BACK MACHINE (alternate-leg version for buttocks and lower back).

STARTING POSITION. Enter the machine from the front by spreading the movement arms. Lie on your back with both legs over the roller pads. Fasten the seat belt and grasp the handles lightly (seat belt should be snug, but not too tight since your back must be arched at the completion of the movement).

MOVEMENT. From the bent-legged position, extend both legs and at the same time push back with your arms. Holding one leg at full extension, allow other leg to bend and come back as far as possible. Stretch. Push out until it joins other leg at extension. Pause and arch your lower back and contract your buttocks. Repeat with the other leg. Important: in the contracted position, you legs should be straight, with knees together, toes pointed.

2. LEG EXTENSION MACHINE (frontal thighs or quadriceps).

STARTING POSITION. In a seated position, place your feet behind roller pads with knees snug against seat. Keep you head and shoulders against seat and lightly grasp handles.

MOVEMENT. Straighten both legs smoothly without jerking. Pause in the contracted position. Slowly lower the resistance to the starting position and repeat.

3. LEG PRESS MACHINE (quadriceps, hamstrings, buttocks).

STARTING POSITION. For best results move quickly from the leg extension to the leg press. Then you pull the seat forward to increase the range of movement. Flip down the foot pads. Place both feet on the pads with toes pointed slightly inward.

MOVEMENT. Straighten both legs in a controlled manner. Return to the stretched position and repeat. Avoid tightly gripping the handles and do not grit teeth or tense face and neck muscles during the movement.

4. LEG CURL MACHINE (back thighs or hamstrings).

STARTING POSITION. Lie face down on the machine. Place your feet under roller pads with your knees just over the edge of the bench. Lightly grasp the handles to keep your body from moving.

MOVEMENT. Curl both legs and try to touch your heels to your buttocks. When your lower legs are perpendicular to the bench, lift your buttocks to increase the movement. Pause at the point of full muscular contraction. Slowly lower resistance and repeat. Important: top of foot should be flexed toward knee throughout the movement.

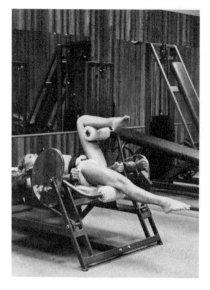

Hip and back machine

Leg extension machine

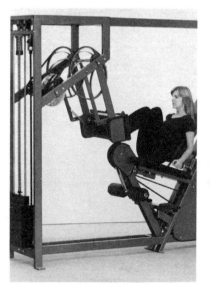

Leg press machine

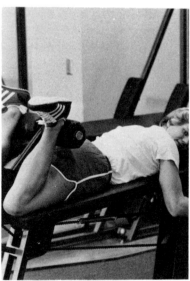

Leg curl machine

5. PULLOVER MACHINE (latissimus dorsi muscles of the back and other torso muscles).

STARTING POSITION. Adjust seat until your shoulder joints are in line with axes of cams. Assume an erect position and fasten the seat belt tightly. Leg press the foot pedal until the elbow pads are about chin level. Place your elbows on the pads with your hands open and resting on the curved portion of the bar.

MOVEMENT. Remove your legs from the foot pedal and slowly rotate your elbows as far back as possible. Stretch, then rotate your elbows (upper arms) down until the bar is on your stomach. Pause, then slowly return to the stretched position and repeat.

6. TORSO-ARM MACHINE (latissimus dorsi of back and biceps of the uppers arms).

STARTING POSITION. First adjust the seat so that you can barely reach the overhead bar. Fasten seat belt. Lean forward and grasp the overhead bar with a parallel grip.

MOVEMENT. Keeping your elbows back, pull the bar behind your neck. Pause. Slowly return to the starting position and repeat.

7. DOUBLE SHOULDER MACHINE

Lateral Raise (deltoid muscles of the shoulders)

STARTING POSITION. Adjust seat so that your shoulders are in line with axes of cams. Fasten the seat belt. Pull handles back until your knuckles touch the pads. Keep your knuckles against the pads and your elbows high at all times.

MOVEMENT. Lead with your elbows and raise both arms until they are parallel with the floor. Hold briefly in the contracted position. Slowly lower the resistance and repeat.

Overhead Press (deltoids and triceps)

STARTING POSITION. With your back flat, grasp the handles above the shoulders.

MOVEMENT. Press the handles overhead. Keep your elbows wide as you slowly lower the resistance. Repeat.

8. NECK AND SHOULDER MACHINE (trapezius and back of neck).

STARTING POSITION. In seated position, place your forearms between the pads. Keep your palms open and back of hands pressed against the bottom pads. Straighten your torso until the weight stack is broken (seat may be raised with elevation pads).

MOVEMENT. Slowly shrug shoulders as high as possible. Pause Slowly return to stretched position and repeat.

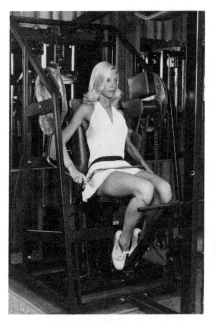

Pullover machine

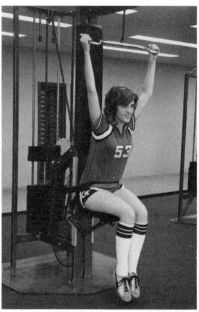

Torso-arm machine

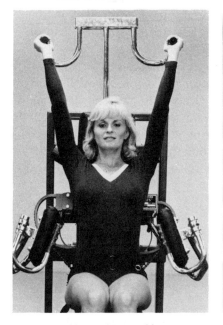

Double shoulder machine

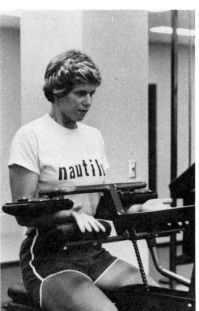

Neck and shoulder machine

9. DOUBLE CHEST MACHINE

Arm Cross (pectoralis majors and deltoids).

STARTING POSITION. Adjust seat until your shoulders (when elbows are together) are directly under the center of the overhead cams. Fasten seat belt. Place your forearms behind and firmly against the movement arms. Lightly grasp the handles (thumb should be around handle) and keep your head against the seat back.

MOVEMENT. Push with your forearms and try to touch your elbows together in front of your chest. Pause. Slowly lower the resistance and repeat.

Decline Press (chest, shoulders, and triceps of arms).

STARTING POSITION. Use the foot pedal to raise handles into starting position. Grasp the handles with a parallel grip. Keep head back and torso erect.

MOVEMENT. Press bar forward in a controlled fashion. Slowly lower the resistance arm while keeping your elbows wide. Stretch at point of full stretch and repeat pressing movement.

10. SQUAT, barbell (thighs, buttocks, and lower back).

STARTING POSITION. In a standing position, the barbell is held and supported across the back of the shoulders. Your feet should be a shoulder-width apart, your back erect, your head up.

MOVEMENT. Lower your body in a controlled manner to a full squat position and smoothly return to the starting position. Take a deep breath and repeat.

11. PULLOVER, barbell plate (torso muscles).

STARTING POSITION. Assume a supine position cross-way on the bench with your shoulders in contact, and your head and lower body relaxed and off the bench. Hold the barbell plate or small dumbbell over you chest in a straight-arm position with thumbs-over grip.

MOVEMENT. Take a deep breath and lower the weight behind your head emphasizing the stretching of the chest and torso. Return to the starting position and repeat.

12. STIFF-LEGGED DEADLIFT, barbell (lower back, buttocks and hamstrings).

STARTING POSITION. The barbell should be grasped with an over and under grip, and smoothly lifted to the standing position.

MOVEMENT. With the knees locked, the barbell is lowered as far as possible and then lifted to the upright position. Repeat.

13. PRESS, barbell (deltoids and triceps).

STARTING POSITION. In a standing position hold the barbell

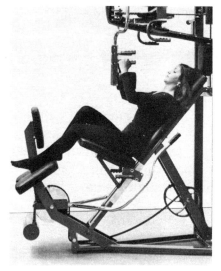

Double Chest 1

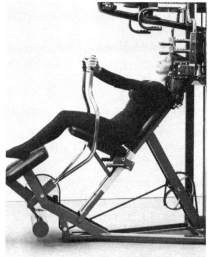

Double Chest 2

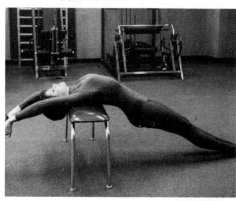

Pullover

Squat

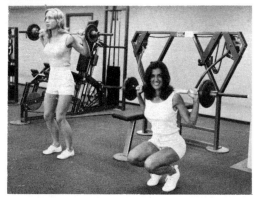

in front of your chest. Your hands should be a shoulder-width apart with your palms facing away from your body.

MOVEMENT. Push the barbell upward until the arms are fully extended over your head. Slowly return to the starting position and repeat.

14. CURL, barbell (biceps of upper arms).

STARTING POSITION. In a standing position, the barbell is held using the palms-up grip with the arms extended at the sides.

MOVEMENT. Curl the weight smoothly until the barbell touches the chest. Slowly lower to the starting position and repeat. Do not "heave" or "throw" the barbell during the movement. Keep your body erect at all times.

15. BENCH PRESS, barbell (chest, deltoids, triceps).

STARTING POSITION. Lying on a bench with connecting supports, you position the barbell with a shoulder-width grip and lift it over your chest.

MOVEMENT. Slowly lower the barbell until it touches your chest, then smoothly press it to a straight-armed position over the chest. Repeat.

16. SHOULDER SHRUG, barbell (trapezius).

STARTING POSITION. In a standing position, the barbell is held with the arms extended.

MOVEMENT. Smoothly shrug your shoulders as high as possible without bending your arms. Pause in the highest position. Slowly lower the barbell and repeat.

17. SIT-UP, accentuate lowering (abdominals).

STARTING POSITION. Anchor your feet under a sturdy object. Your knees should be bent at a 90 degree angle. Raising your buttocks with elevation pads and putting your hands behind your head makes the exercise harder.

MOVEMENT. From a sitting position, slowly lower your torso until your back touches the floor. It should take from six to ten seconds to lower yourself. Once on the floor, use your hands and arms to assist you in the sitting-up process. Important: keep your chin tucked on your chest; keep your shoulders rounded during the movement. Do not arch your back.

18. CHIN-UP, horizontal bar, accentuate lowering (biceps and latissimus dorsi).

STARTING POSITION. For this exercise you will need a small chair or bench to place under the horizontal bar. Step up on

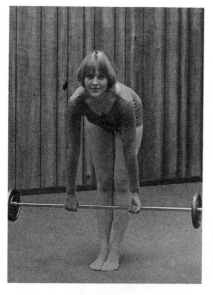

Stiff-legged deadlift

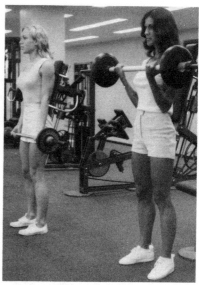

Curl

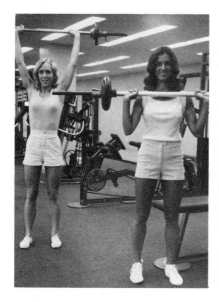

Press

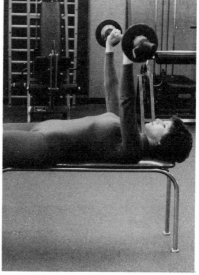

Bench press

the chair and position yourself in a straight-armed position on the parallel bars.

MOVEMENT. Bend your legs, then slowly lower your body between the bars as far as possible. Once again, this should take from six to ten seconds. Return to the starting position and repeat.

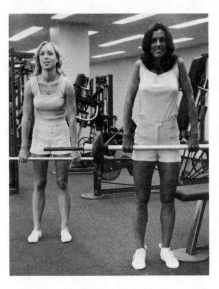

Shoulder shrug

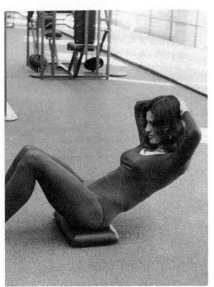

Chin-up

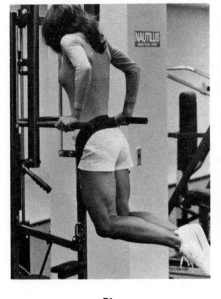

Dip

Sit-up

Dimples, Pockmarks, and Ripples

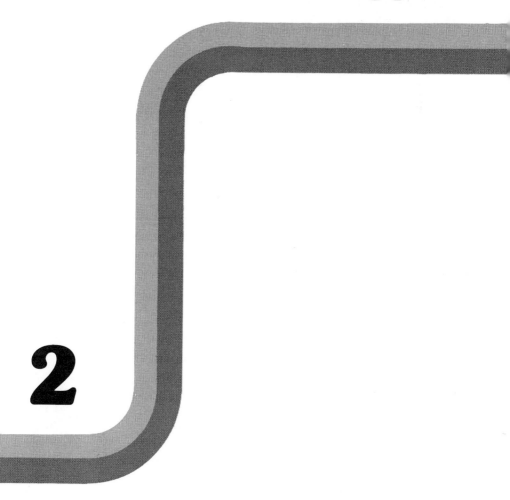

2

DIMPLES, POCKMARKS, AND RIPPLES

"Mirror, mirror on the wall,
Who's the fairest of them all?"

Although your mirror may give its approval as far as facial beauty is concerned, when was the last time you looked at yourself from the rear view? If you are honest in your appraisal, there's a good bet you will not like what you see. Dimples, pockmarks, and ripples in the buttocks and thighs may be the first sign that you are getting out of shape. What started out as pleasing curves may now be a sagging mass of muscle and fat. You can diet until you are blue in the face but it will all be in vain.

Why? The dimple formations and your sagging behind are not the result of an improper diet. They are the result of poor muscle tone. In simple terms, you're spending too much time sitting and not enough time in vigorous exercise. Exercise is the answer to a more shapely posterior. However, the real secret is what kind of exercise and how much. Before specific exercises are discussed, take a good look at the anatomical composition of the buttock area.

ANATOMY OF THE BUTTOCKS

Starting in the middle of the hips and working toward the back, we have a large bone formation called the pelvic girdle. Connecting the pelvic girdle, there are twenty-two major and minor muscles. The most important muscle of this group from the standpoint of buttock shape and size is the gluteus maximus. The major function of this muscle is the extension of the upper leg but only under certain conditions. For example, in easy walking, the muscle remains relaxed and will remain relaxed until you walk very fast, jump, walk upstairs, run, or push something. The general rule seems to be that the gluteus maximus is not called into action in the extension of the upper leg until the hip is flexed in excess of 45%.

Few people are involved in a consistent program of running and jumping once they finish high school. As a result, the dimples and the flabby muscles are just around the corner. Women suffer more than men from this condition partly because their hip widths are greater. The fact that women generally have a higher percentage of body fat than men, does not help the situation either. Women, however, should be aware that the buttocks respond very quickly to progressive exercise.

PROGRESSIVE EXERCISES FOR BUTTOCKS

The exercises that are described in women's magazines may make you more flexible, but they do little to improve your muscle tone. Why? Simply because they are much too easy. The intensity of exercise is much too low. For example, you would have to do literally thousands of side-straddle-hops each day to tone the muscles of your hips.

However, with progressive resistance exercise, all that is needed is one set from eight to twelve repetitions of three basic exercises. For the quickest results, each exercise will be terminated only when no additional movement is possible. This type of training may not be as enjoyable as the so-called "easy exercise" method, but it certainly produces results.

For our purposes, a exercise is progressive only if it involves constantly increasing workloads. The intensity of effort must be increased in proportion to increasing ability, as your muscles become stronger, they must be worked harder. Thus, it is the intensity of exercise that causes the overlying fat and skin to take on new shape and contour.

The recommended exercises for buttocks are listed in three groups. The first group is done with athletic equipment usually found in athletic clubs or spas. This is the fastest and best method of training if you can afford it. The second group can be performed with barbells or dumbbells; and the third group are free-hand exercises.

Group 1 (Nautilus Machines)

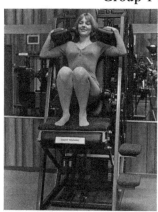

1. Squat machine

Squat machine— This is a compound movement that works the entire lower body: the hips, the thighs, the calves. Photo 1 shows Barbara Simpson at the start of the movement. Barbara has climbed the machine, adjusted the shoulder pads, buckled the seat belt, and is now ready to push the platform down until her legs are straight. She then returns to the starting position and repeats.

31

Geared Hip and Back Machine.----To get to the starting position correctly. Barbara has adjusted her shoulder pads, buckled her retaining

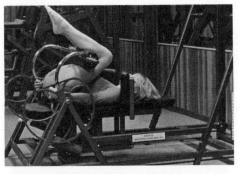

2. Geared Hip and Back

belt, and cranked herself into proper position as shown in photo 2. She then extends her legs by pushing against the rotational movement arm that is located behind the knees. The extension of the upper thighs provides   direct resistance to the buttock muscles as well as those of the lower back. This is the best single exercise for conditioning the hips.

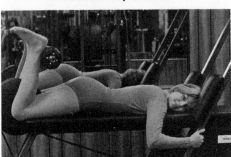

3. Leg Curl

Leg Curl Machine.--- Photo 3 shows Barbara in a contracted position on a Nautilus Leg Curl Machine which exercises the muscles of the thighs and buttocks. The legs are slowly returned to the starting position.

Group 2 (Barbell and Dumbbell)

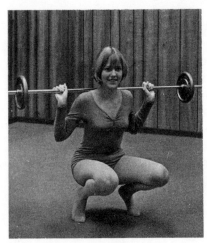

4. Barbell squat

Barbell Squat.--With a barbell securely behind your neck and across your shoulders, bend your legs to a low-squat position as demonstrated in photo 4. Keep your back straight and return to a standing position.

Barbell Deadlift.--- The barbell should be grasped with an overhand grip with the other hand as shown in photo 5(next page) and lifted to a standing position.

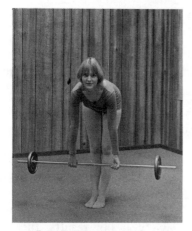

5. Barbell deadlift

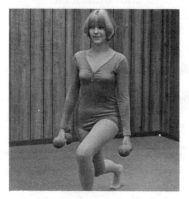

6. Dumbbell lunge

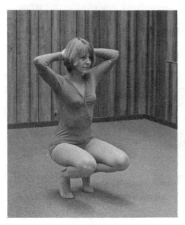

7. Squat

The movement works the hips, the lower back, and the backs of the legs.

Dumbbell Lunge.--- Holding the dumbbell in each hand, you should step forward and bend your leg as shown in photo 6. From this position, bounce up and repeat the process with the opposite leg. Practice getting lower with each repetition. The lunge exercises the thigh and hip muscles.

Group 3 (Freehand Exercises)

Squat.---With your hands on your head, slowly descend to a squat position. You can perform this exercise either flat-footed or on your toes. See photo 7.

Reverse leg raise.--- This is a great free-hand movement for the buttocks. While lying face down and keeping the knees locked, lift both legs as high as possible. Pause briefly at the top position and strongly squeeze the buttock muscles together. Return your legs to the floor and repeat. See the next page for photo 8 of this exercise.

Leg Tuck and Kick.--- From a startting position on your hands and knees, lift one leg and bring your knee and head together as shown in photo 9 (next page). Now straighten and arch your body to the posi-

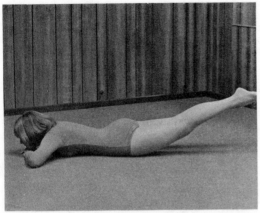

8. Reverse leg raise

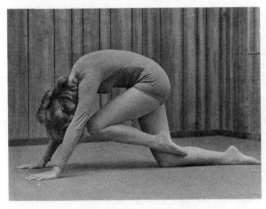

9. Leg tuck and kick

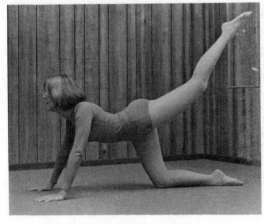

10. Leg tuck and kick

tion in photo 10. Return to the bent-legged position and repeat with the other leg. The back of the thighs and hips are being worked with this movement.

Pick the group of exercises that employs the equipment that is available to you. The free-hand exercises will give you fair results, the barbell and dumbbells will give you better results, and the Nautilus equipment will give you the best results. However, any attempt at conditioning the buttocks will be in vain unless the movements are progressive. A suggested routine would be to start by performing one set of eight repetitions of the three exercises in Group 3. Work out every other day until twelve repetitions are reached. You can now progress to barbell or dumbbell movements (Group 2) or the Nautilus equipment (Group 1). Again, perform eight repetitions on either the barbell or the Nautilus and progress to twelve repetitions. When that many repetitions can be performed in good style, add 5% more resistance and reduce the repetitions to eight.

CONCLUSION

Yes, progressive resistance exercise is the answer to a more shapely figure. Practice the described exercises in the proper manner, and I will guarantee that your "magic mirror" will tell a beautiful story. Say goodbye----FOREVER---- to those dimples, pockmarks, and ripples.

The Answer
to the
Chest-Breast
Quest

3

The Answer To The

CHEST-BREAST QUEST

Remember the story about Don Quixote's quest for the impossible dream? In a similar fashion, I would like to explore one of your dreams and tell you how to make it a reality.

Psychologists inform us that about 95% of the adult population in the United States are dissatisfied with their chest or breast development. Men want to avoid the scrawny or sunken chest look. Women with flat bustlines desire firm, shapely fullness, and those with large breasts are concerned that the "droops" will catch up with them.

While numerous people have wild dreams about their future chest development and spend large sums of money on corrective development, few see their dreams become realities. It is not because their dreams are impossible. Hardly. The fault lies not with the dream, but with the means to that end—the quest.

What is the answer to the chest-breast quest? It should be obvious that the answer is not the latest artificial stimulator, not a wonder cream, and not a revolutionary breast developer.

The answer to a more shapely bust is proper exercise. First, let us take a look at the physiological composition of the chest area. In the center of the chest is the heart which is surrounded by the lungs. The lungs are encircled by the rib cage which connects the backbone to the sternum. The major muscles that surround the back portion of the chest are the latissimus dorsi. The primary muscles of the frontal chest are the pectoralis major which lie on both sides of the sternum. Up to this point the male and female physical makeup is relatively the same.

In addition to the above anatomical description, a mature woman develops breasts in order to supply milk to a newborn infant. While the breasts are attached to the pectoralis major muscles, they are not composed of muscle tissue. Breasts are composed of fatty tissue, glands, and ligaments.

Little can be done to increase the size of the breasts outside of hormone drugs, silicone injections, surgery, or a large decrease or increase in body fat. However, proper exercise can definitely expand the rib cage and increase the size of certain muscle structures. A woman's bustline will take on a new shape and contour as a result of improved strength and tone in the underlying muscles.

Men cannot only improve the tone of the muscles that make up the chest area but also they can develop muscular size and strength that is greater than a woman's. This is mainly because certain hormones are present in greater quanities throughout a man's body.

The primary functions of your chest muscles are to move your upper arms down and across your body. Each recommended exercise performs one or the other of these functions. The exercises for the

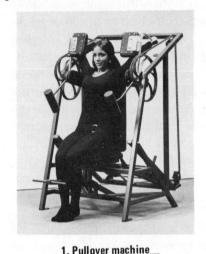

chest are described in three groups. The first group is done with the equipment found in an athletic club or spa. This is the fastest method of training the chest.The second group is performed with barbells and dumbells, and the third group is performed with no special equipment. These exercises are demonstrated by Lynne Pemberton.

Group 1(Using Nautilus Machines)

1. Pullover machine__

Pullover Machine----In order to perform this exercise, sit erect in the seat, fasten the seat belt, and push the foot pedal. The foot pedal moves the elbow pads where they are easily accessible to your upper arms. From the position shown in photo 1, your arms are moved in a rotary fashion until they are slightly behind your waist---photo 2. The pullover exercise provides up to a 240 degree resistance for torso muscles(back, rib cage, chest).

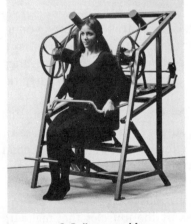

Double Chest Machine--- Two exercises are involved in this machine. The primary exercise is done in alternate arm fashion. The right arm pushes against the elbow pad as the movement arm rotates to the position shown in photo 3 (next page). As your right arm returns the left arm is moved in similar fashion. Direct resistance is provided for the large muscles (pectoralis major) that lie across the

2. Pullover machine

38

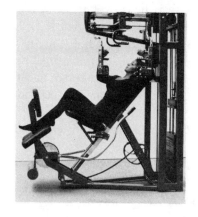

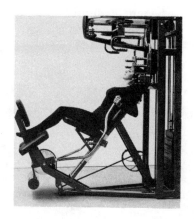

3. Arm cross   **4. Decline press**

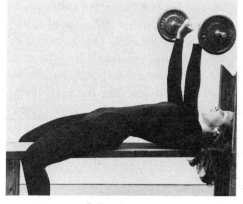

5. Bench press

front of your chest without tiring your arm muscles. The secondary exercise is performed immediately after you have completed the required repetitions of the primary exercise. Photo 4 shows the starting position. From this point, the parallel bars are pushed forward until your arms are straight. The secondary exercise allows you to use the muscles of your arms to force the exhausted chest muscles to work even harder.

Group 2 (barbell and dumbbell)

Bench press — Lying on a bench with support for a barbell, photo 5, the weight is positioned with a shoulder-width grip and arms locked over your chest. Lower the barbell slowly until it touches your chest, photo 6, then push it to a straight-armed position. Your chest, arms. and shoulders are exercised in this movement.

Dumbbell pullover — Assume a supine position cross-way on a bench with shoulders in contact with, and head and lower body relaxed and off the bench. A dumbbell or weight plate is held over the chest in a straight-arm position as shown in photo 7. Take a deep breath, lower the weight behind the head, photo 8, emphasizing the stretching of the torso, and return to a starting position.

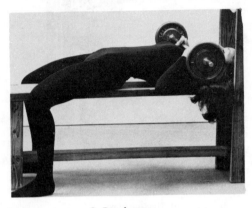

6. Bench press

Group 3(free-hand exercises)

Pushup — When assuming the starting position, be certain your arms are straight, palms flat on the floor. All your weight should be supported by your hands and toes. Slowly bend your arms until your nose touches the floor, then push yourself back to the starting position. If you are not strong enough to do a pushup in this manner, perform it on your knees rather than your toes. You will feel both types in your chest, shoulders, and arms.

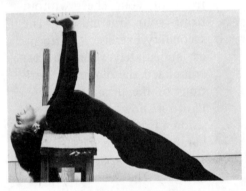

7. Dumbbell pullover (1)

Isometric arm cross—Stand with your arms crossed in front of you and parallel to the floor. Slowly begin to cross your arms harder until an intense contraction is felt. Start gradually using no more than 50% of an all-out effort and gradually build up to a maximum. An isometric contraction should be held about eight seconds with little if any breathing. Breathe deeply before a contraction. Build up

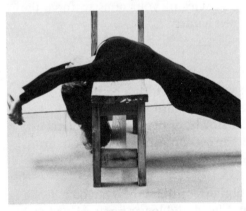

8. Dumbbell pullover (2)

the amount of force for the first three seconds and hold it for at least five. You should feel a strong contraction in the pectoralis muscles where they interlace across the sternum. The isometric arm cross should be done only two times during the workout.

Properly performed, the free-hand exercises will give you fair results, the barbell and dumbbell exercises will give you better results, and the Nautilus machine exercises will give you the best results. However, any attempt at shaping the chests or breasts will be in vain unless the movements are progressive.

For our purposes, an exercise will be progressive only if it involves constantly increasing workloads. The intensity of effort must be increased in proportion to your increasing ability. As muscles become stronger, they must constantly be forced to work harder. Thus it is the intensity of exercise that causes your chest muscles to become stronger and better toned and which causes the overlying breast and skin to take on new shape and contour.

A suggested routine would be to start out by performing one set of eight repetitions of the pushup. Work out every other day, or three times a week, and add a repetition every day until twelve are reached (the isometric arm cross should be performed twice each workout). You can now progress to the barbell and the dumbbell movements (Group 2) or the Nautilus machines (Group 1) if they are available. Again, perform eight repetitions on either the Nautilus machine or barbell and progress to twelve repetitions. When twelve repetitions can be performed in good style, add several pounds and reduce the repetitions to eight.

CONCLUSION

Yes, proper exercise is the answer to the chest-breast quest. In a short time you will be able to walk down the street, take a deep breath, roll back those shoulders, push out that chest, and whistle "The Impossible Dream." You will be the envy of all your friends. Long live Don Quixote!

3 Steps to a Slim, Trim Waistline

4

3 STEPS TO A SLIM, TRIM WAISTLINE

What is the first area of a woman's body to show deterioration? With many women, it is the midsection. Nothing reveals poor physical condition as quickly as a sloppy waistline.

Few things stand out on the beach as much as a slim, trim waistline. Even in clothes a slim waistline can make your positive traits more alluring and your negative ones less noticeable. Witness the current sex appeal of singer-TV personality Cher. Her clothes' designer does everything in his power to emphasize and draw attention to her very muscularly defined waist. Does anyone ever notice that Cher is bow-legged, thin-calved, and slump-shouldered? They are too busy admiring her gyrating navel, etc. Thus, if you want to raise your sex appeal index, knocking off those inches of unwanted flab around the waistline and toning the muscles of the abdomen will boost your stock with men 100%.

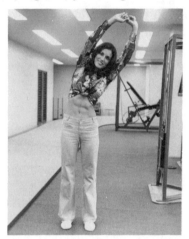

Notice Gayle Barron's slim, trim waistline as she demonstrates the side bend.

Even more important than your appearance is your health. A soft and flabby tummy is good indication that too much fat surrounds your vital organs. Not only does this cause your heart to work much harder than it should, but this condition can possibly lead to other serious ailments.

The following three-step program is designed not only to firm up your waistline, but also to improve you general health. By practicing this routine properly, you can lose several inches from your waist within the next thirty days.

The 3 Steps

1. Posture

One very important fact in slimming your waistline is posture. When the muscle tone of the rectus abdominus decreases through inactivity, the bulging-belly syndrome appears. As muscle tone is lost, the accumulated fat causes the waistline to stretch even further. Poor posture makes the problem worse by accentuating the midsection area. Therefore, lack of tone of the abdominal muscles and poor posture combine to make the waistline sag and bulge. This alone can add two or three inches to your waist measurement.

As a woman becomes overweight, she usually accumulates fat in nature's natural fat storage area which is located in the waist and hip area. This area is called the *panniculus adiposis*. It is a sac-like fat storage area that nature provides us with to be used much the same way a bear stores fat for hibernation. If you were grossly obese, however, the fat would spread to your hips, thighs, chests, arms, and the rest of your body.

2. Diet

To eliminate the fatty tissue around your waist, you must be prepared to reduce the percentage of fat in your body. This simply means you must reduce your daily caloric intake.

The traditionally prescribed 1000-calorie diet was most likely chosen originally by trial and error since its long-term application does produce satisfactory fat loss in all individuals. The actual degree of restriction may be varied according to individual differences between 800 and 1500 calories a day. Here is a sample of a 1000-calorie diet.

1000 Calorie Menu

Breakfast

1/2 cup orange juice
1/2 cup cooked cereal(artificial sweetener may be used)
2 eggs with 1 teaspoon of margarine
1 cup skimmed milk
Black coffee or tea

Lunch

3 ounces lean roast beef
1 slice bread
Green salad as desired
1 medium apple
Coffee or tea

Dinner

1 piece chicken(not fried)
1/2 cup English peas
Green salad as desired
1 slice bread
1/2 banana
1 cup skimmed milk

Such a restricted diet however, must be a balanced diet. It should include one or more servings a day from the Four Basic Food Groups: milk, meat, vegetable-fruit, and bread-cereal groups. It must also include a small amount of fat.

3. Exercise

Exercise is certainly an important factor in slimming your waistline because this improves the muscle tone that in turn tightens the entire midsection area. It also allows you to burn more energy by increasing your metabolic rate. Proper exercise, in combination with the 1000 calorie diet, will guarantee the loss of unwanted flab.

As muscle tone increases from exercise, your posture will also improve. Your midsection will be held flat by the strength of your abdominal muscles; but you will want to help this process by making a concerted effort to sit and stand straight.

The Exercise Routine

As the training director of several athletic clubs, I have used the following three exercises on numerous women with remarkable results. Take a detailed look at each exercise.

Sitting leg tuck. Sit on the edge of a bench or chair, balancing your weight with your hands behind you. Now stretch your legs, point your toes, and raise your feet just above the ground. Bend your knees and try to touch them with your chin(or almost). Then extend or stretch your legs upward at an angle of 45 degrees to the body. Slowly lower your legs to the starting position and repeat.

This exercise works for the entire midsection area, but especially the large rectus abdominus muscles.

Side bend. Stand with your feet slightly apart and link your hands above your head. Bend slowly to the right as far as possible.

Make sure that your arms are held close to your head, that your body does not lean either forward or backward, and that your legs are straight. Return to the starting position and repeat to the left side.

The oblique muscles, located on the sides of your waist, are alternately stretched and contracted in this movement.

Negatively-accentuated sit-up. In the seated position (preferably on a pad) with your feet securely anchored, fold your hands across your chest. While keeping your chin tucked, slowly lower your body (it should take from six to eight seconds) until your back touches the floor. At this point use your hands and arms to assist you in sitting up (so you can concentrate on the lowering or negative position of the

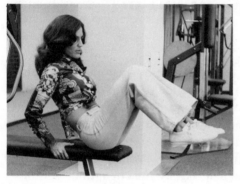

Sitting leg raise

exercise). This is the best single exercise for the muscles that compose the abdominal area.

Generally speaking, most muscle-toning routines should be performed(one set per exercise) three times a week or every other day. Since these exercises will produce muscular soreness in the first week of exercise, I recommend performing the movements six days in a row; during the first week perform all three exercises Monday, Tuesday, Wednesday, Thursday, Friday, Saturday, and exclude Sunday.Then begin your every-other-day program the following Monday. In all instances perform only one set of exercises each training day.In doing the recommended exercises

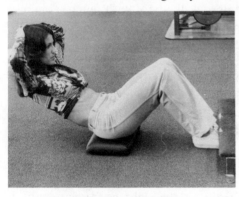

Negative accentuated sit-up

(sitting leg raise, side bend, and the negative-accentuated sit-up), perform eight repetitions the first day. Add another repetition each training day. When twelve can be easily performed, it is now time to make the movements harder. How do you make an exercise harder? There are two ways. You can perform the movements slower or you can increase the resistance.

The slower you perform the movements (up to a point), the better you can concentrate on stretching and contracting the involved muscles. For example, when starting the program, each repetition should take about three to four seconds to perform. As the weeks go by and you get stronger, you can gradually progress to ten to twelve seconds per repetition. When you can perform each recommended exercise for a dozen repetitions in this fashion, you are ready to add resistance.

For additional resistance, you will need several objects (the smaller the better) that weigh approximately 2 1/2, 5, and 10 pounds. Old barbell plates from the garage or basement are ideal, but heavy books or sand bags (plus a little creavity) will work also.

There is no problem in increasing the resistance on the side bend or sit-up. On the side bend you merely hold the weight over your head as you bend. On the sit-up, the weight can be held to your chest, or behind your head (this is the hardest way because of the leverage factor).

On the sitting leg tuck, you will need something to lay across your ankles like an old pair of slacks with knots in the legs. Using this method, you can put a pound or two in each leg and securely lay it across your ankles.

Be sure to stay active on you non-exercise days. Do as much walking as you can. Be conscious of your posture.

Do not forget about the 1000-calorie diet. The recommended exercises will strengthen your midsection muscles, but in order to eliminate the excess fat, you must control your caloric intake.

That is it---posture, weight, and exercise---the three steps to a slim, trim waistline. Give them a thirty day trial. You will not be disappointed.

Building Strength for Tennis

5

BUILDING STRENGTH FOR TENNIS

Have you reached a plateau in your tennis performance? Are your strokes already programmed? Is your tactical knowledge already ingrained? If so, only three, twenty-minute workouts a week of the proper kind of exercise will make you a better tennis player and go a long way toward giving you an advantage over your competition. Interested? Well, read the "why" and "how to."

Picture some of the world's leading tennis players: Jimmy Connors, Chris Evert, Billie Jean King, and Rod Laver.

Do these talented players personify physical fitness and strength to you? Certainly they are tanned, healthy, and superbly skilled and competitive in the sport of tennis. However, Connors and Laver are not physically imposing like football or basketball players of similar esteem. Evert is called "shy and sexy" by some, and Billie Jean has a "chunky" physique with a history of knee problems.

The truth of the matter is: these people are good at tennis in spite of their muscular strength, not because of it. In other words, given stronger muscles, their tennis performance would be even better. Also, a large number of needless injuries could be prevented.

But, more important, the same thing applies to you. That's right! It does not matter if you're a ranked professional, a weekend amateur, or anything in between. If you strengthen the right muscles, I will guarantee that it will improve your tennis game.

How can I make such a guarantee? Although the answer is a bit complex, I think you will understand if you closely follow as I unravel the factors that make up your tennis-playing ability.

Your tennis playing ability is composed of five factors: (1) neurological (brain-nervous system) efficiency, (2) bodily proportions, (3) skill, (4) cardiorespiratory (heart-lung) endurance, and (5) muscular strength.

While each of these factors is important, only one is actually productive. The other four factors are supportive in nature.

Superior neurological efficiency may be almost totally responsible for championship tennis performance if the other four factors are at least average. But neurological efficiency performs no work itself. People with higher levels of neurological efficiency have the ability to contract a larger percentage of muscle mass.

Ideal bodily proportions for tennis are also important for a high level of performance; but again, bodily proportions perform no work of their own. Their contribution to tennis playing consists of providing the working muscles with an advantage in leverage.

Cardiorespiratory endurance is a requirement for life itself, and the lack of it will certainly prevent above average tennis performances. However, no amount of cardiorespiratory endurance will perform work. Movement is produced only by muscular contraction.

Skill is probably the most important factor in tennis performance, but skill alone cannot perform work. What it does do is provide the muscles the ability to work at a higher range of efficiency. It channels the force provided by the muscles in the proper direction, and it helps to prevent a waste of energy involved in an unskilled performance.

All of the first four factors are important in your tennis ability; but none of them do the slightest amount of work. The fifth factor, muscular strength, is the only one that is actually productive. All the others help. They are supportive, but only your muscles perform work.

The first two factors, neurological efficiency and bodily proportions are genetic--determined by heredity-- and are not ordinarily subject to improvement. These factors are either good or bad; but in any case, they are outside our realm of control.

You can do something about the last three factors: skill, cardiorespiratory endurance, and muscular strength. They can be vastly improved.

At the present time, a very high percentage of tennis training is devoted to skill practice; and it should be since skill is probably the single most important factor in tennis playing ability. Cardiorespiratory endurance is also given adequate attention in most tennis training circles; and again, it should be.

Two of our three improvable factors are getting a large amount of attention. One improvable factor--muscular strength--remains largely neglected. It just so happens that muscular strength is the only actually productive one on the list. It is the only factor capable of producing movement, the only factor able to do work.

Well, then, if muscular strength is so important, why is it neglected?

Muscular strength is neglected primarily because it is a feared and misunderstood factor. This misunderstanding is based entirely on superstition, ignorance, and outright fear.

Most tennis players are literally afraid of powerful muscles. Afraid in the sense that they sincerely believe that powerful muscles will somehow limit their performance by reducing their speed of movement and flexibility. In reality, these fears are based on false beliefs that are the exact opposite of the truth.

Stronger muscles will make you faster, not slower, and proper strength training will actually increase your flexibility. Also, greater muscle strength will also go a long way in preventing injuries.

What is proper strength training?

To answer this, we shall have to dig into physiological literature. Once again, the answers are complex; so please bear with me as I try to make them as straight forward as possible.

The basic concepts of strength training were originally tested and defined over thirty years ago by Dr. Thomas DeLorme. They were more recently expanded and updated by Arthur Jones. The cornerstone of strength training, then and now, is PROGRESSION or constantly trying to increase the workload each training session. Progression in exercise is best accomplished with barbells, dumbbells, and weight machines. There is, however, a right and a wrong way to use these exercise tools. Regardless of the training equipment, good results will occur if you apply the following rules.

1. Use as many full range movements as possible to insure the development of the entire length of the involved muscle and to increase flexibility.

2. Perform all repetitions in a rather slow fashion (accentuating the lowering portion of the movement) and avoid throwing or jerking movements.

3. Continue all exercises to a point of momentary muscular failure. This point should be after eight to twelve repetitions working against as much resistance as possible.

4. When twelve repetitions can be performed in good form, add 5% more resistance the next training session and try to perform at least eight repetitions.

5. The entire workout should consist of no more than twelve exercises (four to six for the lower body and six to eight for the upper body); perform only one set of each exercise.

6. Best results occur when there are at least forty-eight hours and not more than ninety-six hours between strength-training sessions.

7. A basic strength-training program for tennis utilizing the Nautilus exercise machines or barbells would look like the following:

Nautilus Machines
Hip and Back
Leg Extension
Leg Curl
Pullover
Double Shoulder
Double Chest
Biceps/Triceps
Wrist-curl on Multi-Exercise
Supination/ Pronation on Sportsmate

Barbell Exercises
Squat
Pullover
Press
Curl
Bench press
Stiff-legged deadlift
Wrist-curl

Over a six-month time period most women should experience strength increases of from 50-100% in all the recommended exercises. Just how much will this improve your tennis? Obviously the answer will vary from individual to individual depending on your age, prior ability, overall potential, and many other factors.

But, in all cases, there will be a measurable degree of improvement; and this improvement will produce a level of performance that you would not have reached without proper strength training.

Remember: a properly conducted strength-training program will not only strengthen your skeletal muscles but will also increase the structural integrity (tendons, ligaments, connective tissue, and bones) of your joints. This will go a long way to the prevention of injuries.

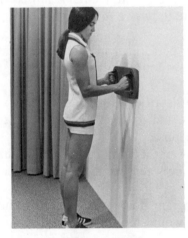

**Supination/Pronation
on Sportsmate**

This exercise is good for prevention of "tennis elbow." Grasp the handles of the unit so that palms face each other. Hold the unit on the wall where your forearms are level with the floor and your elbows form a 90° angle. Keep your elbows at your sides and do not lift them away during the movement. Rotate the right hand and forearm as far clockwise as possible. At the same time resist the clockwise motion with your left arm. Reverse for left arm. To pronate, push instead of twist. Perform 10 repetitions of each.

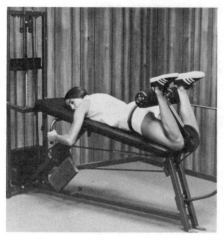

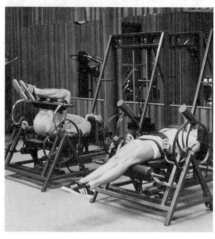

Leg Curl with the hamstrings in full muscular contraction. From this point, the resistance arm is slowly lowered until the legs are straight.

Hip and Back machine provides direct resistance for the large muscles of your buttocks and lower back. Shown are both contracted and stretched position.

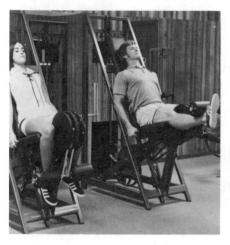

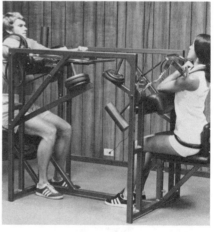

Leg Extension is shown in starting and contracted position. This exercise is good for your frontal thighs.

Biceps/Triceps provides full-range exercise for the upper arms. The contracted position of the triceps is shown on the left side, contracted position of biceps is shown on right side.

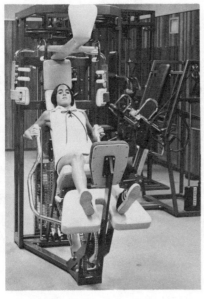

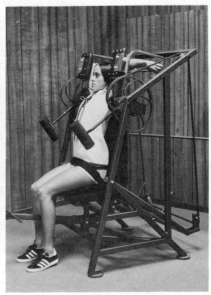

Double Chest (starting position for Decline press) which works on chest, arms, and shoulders.

Pullover machines provide full-range exercises for upper back muscles that are important in tennis strokes.

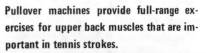

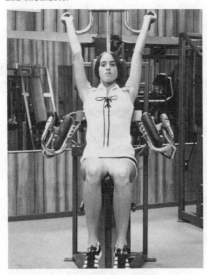

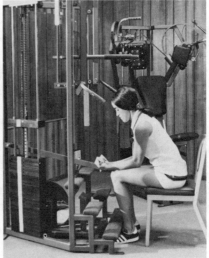

Double shoulder is important to strengthen weak muscles that surround shoulder girdle. Especially good for women.

Wrist curl on Multi-Exercise machine. Stabilize forearms and elbows on thighs. Curl handles smoothly, first underhand grip, then overhand grip.

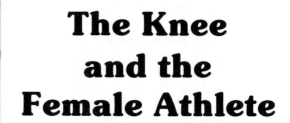

The Knee
and the
Female Athlete

6

THE KNEE AND THE FEMALE ATHLETE
Ouch . . .Ow . . .Snap . . .Crackle . . .Pop
go the knees!

The useful, abused, stubborn, delicate, sexy knees. They can be dimpled, bony, knobby, knocked, bowed, gnarled, cute, or sturdy as an oak.

Versatile? Yes ma'm. You close a stuffed suitcase with the pressure of a knee. You show reverence to royality by planting a knee on the carpet. Your scrub the kitchen floor on your knees. You plug in the electricity while on your knees. You crawl on your knees. You flirt with your knees. You even use them as weapons.

Vulnerable? That too. Last year in the United States over 63,000 knee injuries attributed to sports required surgery. Everyone has read about Joe Namath's knees. But did you know that Billie Jean King and Maria Bueno have had knee operations?

Knee injuries are amazingly common among women, especially teenage girls. Why? Primarily for three reasons: (1) the wider female pelvis angles the thigh bones into the joint more sharply, increasing the stress on the knee, (2) the beginning of the female hormonal flow seems to relax the ligaments in preparation for child-bearing, (3) lack of strength (or disproportional strength) in the large muscles that surround the knee joint. The first two reasons, plus the lack of strength, make the knee particularly vulnerable to sharp turns in field hockey and basketball, and sudden stopping and starting on the tennis court, and a host of other skills that involve running, jumping, and body contact.

Little or nothing can be done about the first and second reasons for injury. However, the third cause, muscular strength, can definitely be improved. Proper strength training of thigh and calf muscles can go a long way toward providing maximum knee protection for females.

Before strength-training exercises are discussed, let us take a close look at the anatomy of the knee. If you have a small understanding of the knee joint—its weak and strong points—you should be better qualifed to protect it from injury.

Anatomy of the Knee
The knee joint is the largest joint in the body and from an architectural point of view one of the weakest. Its architectural weakness is due to the fact that in no position of flexion or extension are the bones involved in the joint ever in more than partial contact. This is of

special interest to athletes because your knees support your entire weight; and stopping and starting movements put tremendous pressure. on the knee joint.

The knee is essentially a hinge,or movable joint held together by a system of tendons and ligaments. In fact , there are thirteen distinct ligaments that enter into its strength and support.

A small bone in front of the joint is the patella, or knee-cap, which is attached by the patellar tendon to the quadriceps (frontal thigh muscles) and to the surface of the tibia (lower leg bone). The pressure of the femur (thigh bone) on the tibia is cushioned by a set of cartilage pads (menisci) that fit the uneven bony surfaces of the knee.

The knee's hinge motion is accompanied by a small amount of external and internal rotation. The knee is best, however, at forward and backward flexion and extension. Try to do other movements with your knee and you may have problems.

Most knee injuries among male athletes occur when the foot is firmly planted on the ground and a strong force (like a fast moving athlete) whams against the joint. For example, this may happen when a quarterback is back to pass and is blind-sided by a tackler.

Women tennis players, skiers, golfers, basketball players, and even joggers can be similarly injured with their body-weight providing the necessary force. Perhaps your foot "catches" and you stumble foward twisting the knee as you fall.

Usually the ligaments of the knee bear the brunt of the dammage. The damage can range from a simple stretching of the colateral ligaments, usually on the inner side of the knee, to a partial or complete tear of the ligament to a severe three-part injury that includes a rupture of the collateral ligament on the inner side of the knee, a shredding of the meniscus (cartilage) as it is ground between the twisting bones, and a rupture of the anterior cruciate ligament. The three-part injury calls for immediate surgery and sidelines the athlete for the season.

The menisici or knee cartilages, whose function is not completely understood, are a common source of knee trouble. Even when you kneel or twist your knee, the cartilage may be squeezed out of its normal position in the joint. As a result, the meniscus may catch in the joint and tear. Menisci lack a blood supply and do not heal; so a torn fragment may interfere with smooth operation of a joint, causing it to lock painfully unless the fragment is removed.

The Knee and the Female Athlete

Some of the most significant advances with knee injuries have been in diagnostic techinique. Doctors once were handicapped in assessing knee damage because neither ligament nor cartilage register on X ray. Now a contrast media can be injected that makes tissue stand out so that injuries can be detected.

Even more dramatic, a lighted magnifiying scope, the diameter of a pencil point, can be inserted in certain cases and the physician can actually see how the knee has been injured. For more routine cases, a tap of knee fluid is taken. Clear fluid indicates that no ligaments are torn. The presence of blood in the fluid usually indicates a ligament injury. Fat in the fluid indicates a fracture.

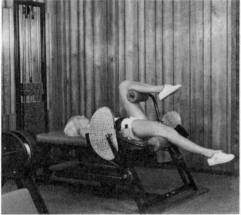

Hip and back, stretched position

Torn cartilage removal is a common, but still controversal, operation. Advocates say it can restore almost complete function of the knee. Others note that persons who have had cartilage removed are more likely to have degenerative arthritis in later years. In any case, the removal of shattered cartilage is often a must if the knee is to remain fully functional. Cartilage removal does not require a very long period of immobility. A padded bandage is worn for a few weeks, and this is followed by several months of exercise to regain muscular control of the knee. A minor knee injury, like a simple stretching of the collateral ligament, usually heals with a few days' rest and an elastic bandage for support. It is true that a partially torn ligament must

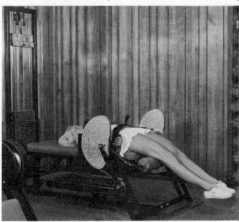

Hip and back, contracted position

be immobilized by strapping or by encasing the knee in a plastic case for up to three weeks, with the victim on crutches. A rupture of one or more ligaments requires surgery as soon as possible. Within a few days after the initial injury, the ligaments begin to shrivel and cannot be rejoined properly.

Surgery for serious knee injuries (ruptured ligaments) calls for total immobilization in a hip-to-foot cast for six to eight weeks, but the knee can be restored to full use in most cases, especially if proper rehabilitative exercises are followed.

Strength Training for the Knee

Although many of today's athletes have the best in modern medicine and surgical science to help them recover from knee injuries, the area of prevention has almost been ignored. One well-known sports doctor even goes so far as to say that 50% of all knee injuries could be prevented by proper strength-training and conditioning. Even if injury could not have been prevented, it makes sense that the stronger the leg muscles, the better they will withstand force; and the less severe injury will be.

The strength of the thigh and calf muscles offers the first line of defense against the stress received by an athlete's knee. High levels of strength in the thigh and calf muscles can be obtained by performing one set of four to six leg exercises, using Nautilus or conventional exercises three times a week.

NAUTILUS MACHINES	BARBELLS/OTHERS
1. Hip and Back	1. Squat
2. Leg Extension	2. Leg extension
3. Leg Press	3. Leg press
4. Leg Curl	4. Leg curl
5. Calf Raise	5. Calf raise

Perform the recommended five exercises in the high-intensity fashion (eight to twelve repetitions) with special emphasis on good form. Remember, it should take approximately two seconds to smoothly raise the resistance and four seconds to smoothly lower the resistance.

Over a six-month period of time most female athletes will see strength increases of from 50-100% in all the recommended exercises. For example, take the leg extension exercise, during the first week of training, you successfully perform ten repetitions with forty pounds

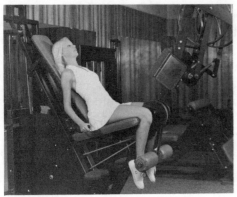

Leg extension, starting position

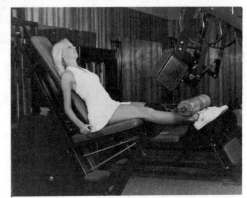

Leg extension, contracted position

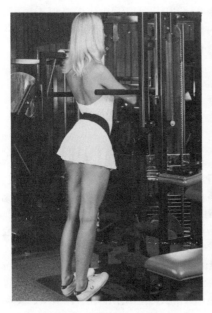

Calf raise, stretched position

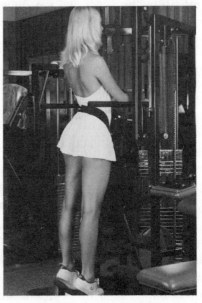

Calf raise, contracted position

of resistance. Six months later, after training three times a week, you perform ten repetitions with eighty pounds. Practically speaking, you have increased your leg-extension 100%. Similar increases are possible in the other exercises.

A properly conducted strength-training program will not only strengthen your skeletal muscles (the first line of defense against injury), but will also increase your structural intregrity (tendons, ligaments, connective tissue, and even bones) of your joints. This will go a long way toward the the prevention of many sports- related injuries, not to mention the improved performance that results when your muscles become stronger.

Other factors related to knee injuries should also be mentioned. These are:

Unequal leg strength--80% of the knee injuries occur on the weak leg side of the body. Thus, special attention should be given to strengthening the weak leg. Many two-legged exercises can be performed one-legged to make sure that the strong leg is not favored (leg extension, leg curl, leg press).

Leg length inequalities--- Many athletes have minor inequalities in the length of their legs (usually under one inch) that can be measured as well as observed. If knee injuries happen to these people, careful study shows that the injury occurs about 88% of the time to the short leg. These lateral inbalances can be corrected during a child's growing period. Later in life one should wear a built-up shoe.

Lack of ligament stability--Youngsters with hyperextension of the knee joint are particularly prone to injury. This condition has a very unstable effect on the knee. In these cases considerable attention should be given to the development of the hamstrings as well as the medial and lateral components of the musclar support.

Faulty movement mechanics--Athletes should be encouraged to walk and run in a pigeon-toed manner. This action aids in the stability of the inside of the knee as well as preventing the external rotation of the tibia (beyond the normal) in cutting and turning.

Poor off-season training--Close to 75% of all types of sports' injuries occur during the first two weeks of practice. This is probably due to the fact that most athletes do not maintain first-class conditioning during the off season. Be sure to have both an in-season and off-season conditioning program.

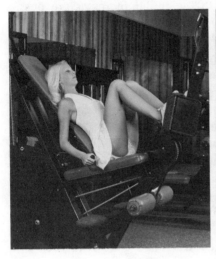

Leg press, starting position

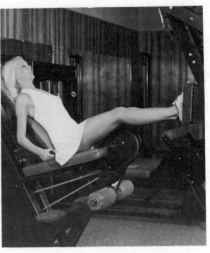

Leg press, finishing position

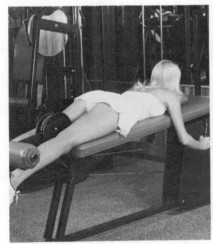

Leg curl, starting position

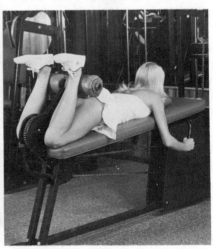

Leg curl, contracted position

The Knee and the Female Athlete

Guidelines to Follow When an Injury Occurs

When an injury occurs to the knee, first-aid treatment should be initiated immediately. If possible, a wet elastic wrap should be applied to the area with minimum delay. The wet wrap is used to apply pressure and quickly conduct the cold from an ice pack to the injured area. An icepack (a wet towel full of ice chips or a chemical cold pad) is then applied. The ice pack is held in place with a dry plastic wrap and the knee is elevated. The cold treatment should be carried out at thirty to forty-five minute intervals in the forty-eight hours following an injury.

An elastic wrap should be applied to control the swelling and support the joint. If the injury is moderate to severe, crutches should be used and an orthopedic specialist consulted.

Upon clearance from the physician, treatment and therapy should be started. Regaining the normal range of motion of the joint and continuing to control swelling are the goals of the initial treatment.

Ice massage is one therapeutic agent that may be used. A seven ounce paper cup is filled with water and placed in the freezer. When frozen, apply the ice cup—gradually peel the cup away— in small circular motions to the injured area. This should be done for eight minutes. Four sensations will occur during the application: cold, burning, throbbing, and numbness. When the area is numb, three minutes of exercise should be performed.

The exercise should consist of attempting to flex and extend the knee through its full range of motion. This is followed by eight more minutes of ice, three more minutes of exercise, eight ice, three exercise. Use this combination of ice and exercise in the three sets just mentioned, three times a day.

Whirlpool treatment may be used. A low temperature—50-60 degrees F— should be used at first for fifteen minutes a day. The low water temperature discourages swelling in the area. The temperature should be slowly increased until a temperature of 104 degrees F is reached. At this temperature the time should be fifteen minutes also. Be sure and perform flexion and extension movements at the knee joints while standing in the whirlpool.

Rehabilitation

Although some rehabilitation should occur at the time of injury, a more vigorous, active rehabilitation starts when the athlete exhibits a normal range of movement with the injured knee. The muscles that cross the knee-joint must be strengthened to provide stability to the injured joint. Because these muscles are very large, a great degree of strength can be developed in this area, and the joint can be conditioned to be extremely stable to prevent reoccurance of the injury. A progressive program should be initiated. When the exercise can be executed with no pain, the activity should be intensified.

Weight equipment should be utilized for rehabilitation purposes. Three sets of eight to twelve repetitions at a comfortable weight is recommended. Weighted boots or commercial exercises machines designed specifically for knee rehabilitation may be used. The Nautilus Leg Extension and Leg Curl Machines are by far the best on the market.

Lateral leg raises from a standing position are also recommended. Do twenty repetitions at a time, three times a day. One-legged calf raises are also beneficial; do three sets of twelve repetitions. However, if pain occurs throughout any phase of rehabilitation, work with lighter loads or do less repetitions.

As you progress, light jogging may be started in a straight-line pattern. The knee should be supported with an elastic bandage to prevent swelling in the area. Absorbant, rubber-soled shoes should be worn. After a while you may gradually progress to running that involves a change in direction.

Returning to Competition

The goal of your rehabilitation program should be bilateral equality of leg strength and antagonistic muscle balance. Both legs should measure approximately the same at the mid calf, knee cap, two inches above the knee, and seven inches above the knee cap. Equal leg strength—right vs. left leg— should be displayed in the leg extension and leg curl exercises. A person should be able to run figure eight and circular patterns of decreasing size without pain or limp. Adhesive strapping or bracing of the knee is not necessary if the knee is properly rehabilitated and if conditioning continues throughout the season. Time and expense in utilizing tape can be avoided if a sound rehabilitation program is followed.

It is most important to remember that strength training is the prime defense against injury, and the muscles that cross the knee joint must be strengthened and conditioned preseason. This conditioning should be continued throughout the season to insure freedom from injury. If an injury does occur , proper rehabilitation is essential in returning the athlete to activity and avoiding reoccurance.

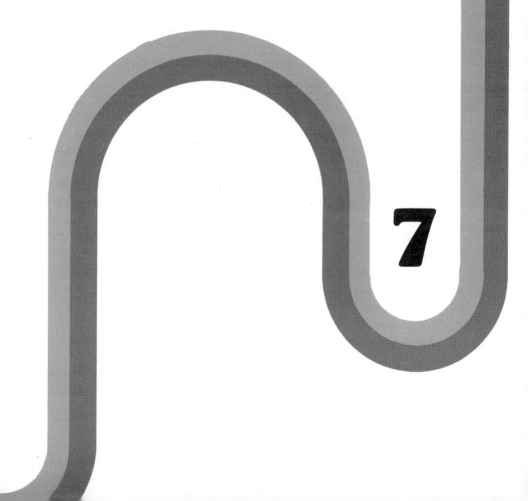

Strength Training
for the
Over 50 Age Group

7

STRENGTH TRAINING FOR THE OVER 50 AGE GROUP

*If you suffer from stiff joints and would like
to remedy the situation, the following information
can be of great value to you.*

Have you ever noticed that many elderly people develop that stiff shuffle with hunched shoulders? These characteristics can be eliminated if the major muscles of the body are properly strengthened.

Is muscular strength really important for the over 50 age group? Definitely--- and for several good reasons.

First, strength is the major component of all physical activities, because, muscles, by contracting and relaxing, move our bodies. Our entire movement potential, in fact, is controlled by skeletal muscles. The stronger your muscles are, the more efficiently you move.

Second, a muscle that has been strengthened properly is also more flexible. Not only should your muscles be contracted, they should also be stretched. It is the stretching movement that increases your flexibility. The stretching is made possible by resistance that is heavy enough to smoothly push or pull the involved body part into a position that actually exceeds your momentarily existing range of movement.

Third, strong muscles offer the first line of defense against injury. They give you protection from force--whether it be from a fall, from an automobile accident, or from a mugger. Proper strength training strengthens your ligaments, tendons, connective tissue, and even bones. It has been proven that proper exercise provides linear stress to the bones, which helps to prevent osteoporosis (porous bones) and osteomalciar (soft bones).

A properly conducted strength-training program will benefit all men and women, especially the over fifty age group. But, let me caution you, it must be proper strength training. Just any exercise will not do the job. How you do the exercise is as important as which exercise you do.

Before starting the strength-training program, be sure and get the approval of your personal physician. He will probably want to give you a thorough physical examination that includes a cardiological stress test.

Basic exercises should be selected to involve major muscle groups. Where a choice exists, such exercises should involve the greatest possible range of movement. If the proper selection of exercises is made, then only a few movements are required to improve your strength and overall muscle tone.

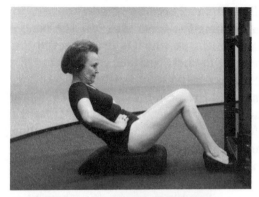

Sit-ups------good for your stomach. Keep your head and shoulders rounded as you lower yourself. Always use your arms to help you back to starting position.

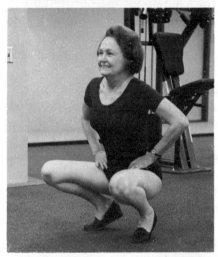

The squat or deep-knee bend is an all-around exercise for the lower body. Keeping your back erect, slowly descend to a full squat. It is okay to have help returning to the standing position.

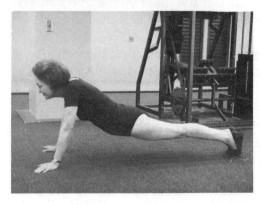

In the push-up, use your knees and lower back to get you in the starting position shown. Slowly bend your arms in a controlled fashion. When you reach the floor, assist yourself with your knees once again. Repeat.

Strength Training for the Over 50 Age Group

What exercises are best for the over fifty age group? Nautilus machine exercises are especially beneficial because you do not have to involve the hands and arms in working the torso muscles. The Nautilus machine also provides rotary resistance which is very important in increasing your flexibility. Some of the best Nautilus exercises are hip and back extension, leg curl, leg extension, pullover, shoulder shrug, neck extension and flexion, and neck rotation.

Barbell exercises can also be used effectively. The best barbell exercises are the squat, stiff-legged deadlift, standing press, standing curl, and stiff-armed or bent-armed pullover.

Other barbell and free-hand exercises that are of value—but are not as productive as those previously listed— are the shoulder shrug, bench press, calf raise, wrist curl, the chin-up on the horizontal bar (palms-up grip), the dip on the parallel bars, and the free-hand squat, push-up, and sit-up.

Perhaps you would like to get started on a strength-training program but there is no equipment. What do you do?

First, select several large muscle exercises that require no special equipment. The free-hand squat, the push-up, and the sit-up are good ones. With a little creativity you should be able to rig up a chinning bar and some type of parallel bars.

Start out by performing eight repetitions of each exercise in good form. That may seem impossible on some movements, especially the chin-up, dip, and even push-up. If that is the case, here is what to do.

In the chin-up, you can use your legs to get your chin over the bar. Simply place a wooden box or chair in front of the chinning bar and step on the box, rather than pulling up with the arms, until your chin is over the bar. Remove your feet and lower yourself very slowly, six to eight seconds. Climb back and repeat. It is a great exercise for arms and back muscles.

Remember, for building strength, research has shown that the lowering portion of the exercise is far more important than the raising portion.

Dips on the parallel bars can be done in a similar fashion. Climb up, lock your arms, your arms should be about a shoulder-width apart, and lower your body very slowly. This exercise works the chest, shoulders, and triceps. If you are unable to perform a dip in this manner, try the push-up.

In the push-up, use your knees and lower back to help straighten your arms. Then, slowly bend your arms until your chest touches the floor and repeat.

For stomach strength, do sit-ups in the same (accentuate the lowering) fashion. With the knees bent, feet securely held down, and hands on your waist, slowly lower your upper body until your back touches the floor. It is important to keep your chin tucked and shoulders rounded throughout the lowering. Once on the floor, use your arms to assist in the sitting-up movement.

The squat can be performed in the following way: with your hands on your hips and your back erect, slowly bend your knees and descend to the full-squat position. It should take about ten seconds for you to properly lower yourself. Stand up quickly and repeat. You may use a chair or support of some type to assist you in standing up.

For best results from these movements, only one set of eight to twelve repetitions, three times a week, should be done.

These five exercises—-squat, chin-up, dip, sit-up, push-up—done in the accentuate-the-lowering fashion, should form your beginning strength-building program. After using these exercises for several months, you can gradually add a few barbell exercises or Nautilus machine exercises, if Nautilus machines are available.

If you are going to use the barbell exercise program, be sure to spend the first couple of workouts practicing the movements with nothing more than an empty bar (most bars weigh from fifteen to twenty pounds). Stress correct form in all exercises: two seconds in the lifting phase and four seconds in the lowering phase. Remember: fast movements are very dangerous. Every movement should be performed smoothly.

At the beginning of any strength-training, muscle-toning program, correct form should be emphasized much more than other factors. Without proper form, your workouts become meaningless.

In organizing and starting a strength-training program, be conscious of the following rules:

1. Select exercises that involve large muscle groups throughout a great range of movement.

2. Stress correct form.

3. Emphasize the lowering portion of all exercises.

4. Perform eight to twelve repetitions.

5. Train three times a week.

6. As time goes by, gradually work up in the concepts of progression and intensity (see article 1 for a complete description of progression and intensity).

7. Under all circumstances get the approval of your personal

physician before starting the program.

REMEMBER: strength training can enrich the well-being of all women and men. It can increase your muscular strength and flexibility. It can improve your posture and gait. It can protect you from injury. But, it must be proper strength training— properly organized, properly supervised, and properly performed.

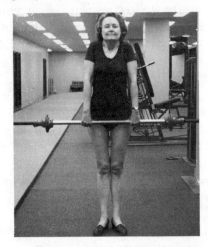

On the left is the shoulder shrug. Try to raise your shoulders as high as possible without bending your arms. Good for the upper back.

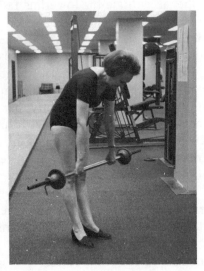

The photo on the right shows the stiff-legged deadlift. It is a good exercise to contract the hamstring, buttock, and lower back muscles.

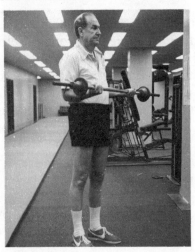

On the left is the barbell curl which is a good way to strengthen and condition bicep muscles. Let your arms lift the barbell, not your legs or lower back.

NAUTILUS MACHINE EXERCISES

1. PULLOVER MACHINE. Notice on page 72 Pat Peterson uses this machine for increasing the strength and flexibility around her shoulders. For best results, be sure and do this movement in a slow deliberate manner.

2. 4-WAY NECK MACHINE. Posterior extension for the head and the back of the neck is demonstrated by George Peterson. This machine can also be used to work the front and the sides of the neck.

3. MULTI EXERCISE MACHINE. Mr. Peterson demonstrates the **DIP** in this picture. To perform this exercise, climb up until you are able to lock you arms (use a small chair bench to step up on) and slowly lower yourself by bending your arms. You will feel this one in your shoulders, chest, and arms.

Follow a similar procedure in performing the **CHIN-UP.** Step up on a chair and place your chin over the horizontal bar. Now slowly lower your body to a dead hang. Keep repeating until you are no longer able to control your descent. Your arms and back are working in this movement.

Lack of strength and flexibility in the calf and ankle is a major problem in the over 50 age group. Much of this can be eliminated by properly performing the **CALF RAISE** on the **MULTI-EXERCISE NAUTILUS** machine. Keeping your knees locked, slowly lower your heels as far as possible while balancing on the balls of your feet. Stretch. Now raise your heels and stand on your toes and once again lower your heels.

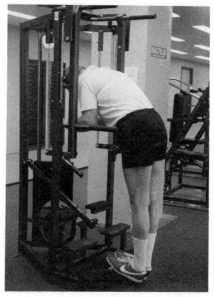

C a l f   r a i s e

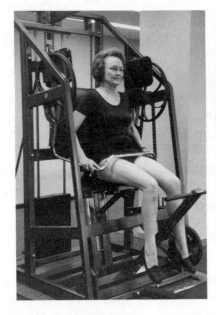

1. Pullover

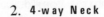

2. 4-way Neck

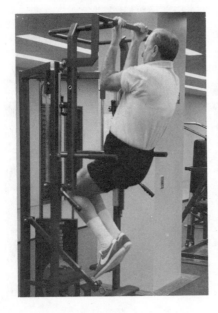

3. Chin-up

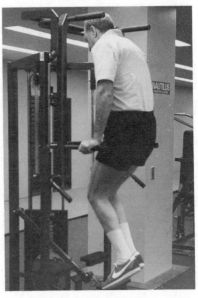

4. Dip

Something for Men:
Questions and Answers about
Muscle and Fat

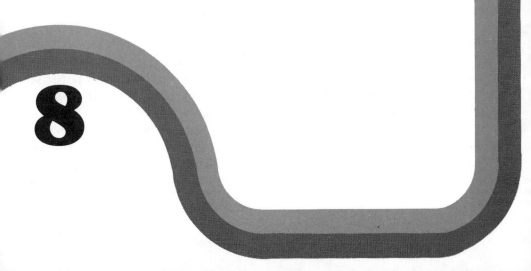

8

SOMETHING FOR MEN:
QUESTIONS AND ANSWERS ABOUT MUSCLE AND FAT

Muscle and fat are two essentials of the human body. Yet these two important elements are often misunderstood when the subject of exercise is discussed.

The human body contains three types of muscles: the voluntary or skeletal muscles, the involuntary muscles such as those of your digestive tract, and the heart muscle. In exercise we are primarily concerned with the skeletal muscles, because when these muscles contract, our body moves.

Our movement potential is brought into action by over four hundred and thirty-four skeletal muscles. They are composed of two hundred and fifty million smaller units, the muscle fibers, and make up 40% of the body weight of the typical American male.

On the other hand, at least 20% of the average man's body weight is in the form of fat---or adipose tissue. The major function of fat is long-term storage of energy. Additional functions are to provide heat and protection for the body and inner organs. Fat, though, does not contribute to muscular contraction. In fact, fat between muscle fibers acts as a friction brake and can actually impede the normal relatively frictionless movement of the lean muscle fibers during exercise.

In most sports muscles contribute almost everything while fat contributes nothing. As a result, millions of dollars are spent each year by coaches and athletes (as well as the general public) on muscle-building and fat-reducing programs. Most of these, unfortunately, are worthless. Even if a program has merit, much of the possible results are usually neglected or lost due to misconceptions about training.

It would be wise to answer some of the most frequently asked questions about muscle and fat. Correct answers to these questions can help you eliminate misconceptions and greatly improve your own training program.

WHAT MAKES MUSCLES GROW?

Muscle growth consists of two parts. One, there must be growth stimulation within the body itself at the basic cellular level. After puberty, this is best accomplished by high-intensity exercise. Two, the proper nutrients must be available for the stimulated cells. Large amounts of nutrients, in excess of what your body needs, will not do anything to promote the growth of muscle fibers. The growth machinery within the cell must be turned on first. Muscle stimulation MUST always precede nutrition. If you have stimulated muscular growth by high-intensity exercise, then your muscles will grow with almost any reasonable diet.

The chemical reactions inside growing muscles are much more complicated than just exercising and eating. High-intensity muscular contraction results in the formation of a chemical called creatine. The creatine stimulates the muscle to form myosin, one of the contraction proteins within the muscle fiber. Thus, contraction of the muscle fibre produces creatine, which in turn causes the muscle to form more myosin, which enables it to undergo more contractions. This, in turn, causes the production of more creatine; and around we go again.

Creatine has been identified as the messenger substance that turns on the RNA (ribonucleic acid) processing line to produce muscle growth. The RNA within a specialized compartment of the cell literally acts like an assembly line and hooks together various combinations of amino acids, sometimes in combination with complex sugars and fats, to form different compounds that result in the increased size of certain muscle cells. Remember: first, you stimulate growth through high-intensity exercise; then, you must provide the proper nutrients.

WHAT DO YOU MEAN BY HIGH-INTENSITY EXERCISE?

For our purposes, high-intensity exercise means the repetitive performance of a resistance movement that is carried to the point of momentary muscular failure. Generally this means that one set of each exercise should be performed in strict style for ten repetitions. At least eight repetitions should be performed and not more than twelve. If you cannot make eight, then the resistance is too heavy; and if you can perform more than twelve, the resistance is too light.

The real key to this technique is "pushing" yourself, or being pushed by someone else, to perform as many strict repetitions as possible. A set is considered finished when it is momentarily impossible to perform another full repetition.

When you can perform twelve repetitions, add a small amount of resistance--about 5% more-- and reduce the repetitions to eight. Try to add an additional repetition each training day. Always add weight when you can perform twelve or more repetitions in good form.

WHAT IS GOOD FORM?

Good form requires all the repetitions to be executed in a slow, smooth style. No throwing or jerking movements should be practiced. It is important that special attention be given to lowering the resistance (eccentric contraction). Research shows that for building muscular size and strength, lowering the resistance is much more important than raising the resistance. For example, if it takes two seconds to raise a weight, it should take four seconds to lower the same weight. All in all, it should take about one minute to complete a set of ten repetitions in good form.

WHERE DOES PRE-STRETCHING FIT IN PROPER FORM?

Pre-stretching is involved when a muscle is pulled into a position of increased tension prior to the start of the contraction. When a muscle is pre-stretched, a neurological signal is sent to the brain that results in a higher percentage of the muscle being contracted.

All athletes consciously and unconsciously use pre-stretching in some fashion to their advantage. Take the baseball hitter who swings before he hits the ball, or the boxer who draws back his fist before a punch, or the shot-putter who gets that little dip just before he throws.

Pre-stretching can be used effectively in strength-training sessions. Practiced properly, you will be able to handle heavier weights and thus bring into an action a greater percentage of your muscle mass during each repetition. There is a thin line, however, between (1) pre-stretching a muscle in the starting position of an exercise and following through with the repetition in the proper manner, and (2) pre-stretching a muscle in the starting position and throwing the resistance. The key points to remember are: pre-stretch---move quickly---and then slow down.

In other words, the weight should be lowered from the contracted position in a controlled manner until the bar or the resistance arm is about one inch from the position of full stretch. At that point, there should be a very quick twitch or thrust. After the quick twitch, the movement should be slowed down in a controlled manner. The only time the bar or resistance arm should be moved quickly is during the first one-quarter to one-half of the raising (positive) part of the repetition. The last half of the repetition should always be performed smoothly.

WHY IS HIGH–INTENSITY EXERCISE BEST FOR STIMULATING MUSCULAR GROWTH?

High-intensity exercise is best for several reasons. First, it is by far the safest way to train. Training injuries occur when a muscle exerts a force that exceeds the breaking strength of some part of the muscular structure. By performing ten repetitions, as opposed to heavy maximum attempts, the intensity is high and the force is low.

Second, high-intensity exercise produces faster results from less training time. Ten sets of any exercise terminated two repetitions short of a point of momentary failure will not produce results anywhere close to those that can be produced by one properly performed set carried to a point of failure. When you increase the intensity of an exercise, your amount of exercise must be reduced. A full routine for the major muscles of the body can be completed in less than thirty minutes. Training properly, it is not uncommon for the average man to double his overall body strength in less than a year.

Third, high-intensity training makes less demands upon your recovery ability than traditional training methods. Recovery ability is related to your system as a whole. Long, grueling workouts constantly force your recovery ability to work as hard as possible merely to replace the large amount of energy expended. As a result, very little is left as a reserve for growth and strength increases.

High-intensity training and a large amount of training are mutually exclusive programs. You can have one or the other but never both. Therefore, for stimulating muscular growth, practice your exercise in a high-intensity fashion, but keep it brief and frequent.

WHY DOES FAT TEND TO ACCUMULATE AROUND MY WAIST?

There are individual tendencies to develop a high density of fat-storage cells in different body areas. This is an inherited characteristic that cannot be altered. Some people naturally accumulate noticeable fat on their legs and hips, others on their back and neck; but generally speaking, most people (especially men after the age of thirty), tend to store fat around the waist.

The average male college student has approximately 18% of his body weight in the form of fat, and the average female college student has about 26%. About half of the body fat is right under the skin, and a large portion of the other half is around your inner organs. Most authorities think for optimum performance, an athlete should have 12% or less body fat.

HOW CAN I REDUCE MY PERCENTAGE OF BODY FAT?

In order to reduce your percentage of body fat, you have to force your body to burn its own fat as a source of energy. To do this, you must keep your caloric intake below your maintenance level. Consuming one thousand less calories a day than your maintenance level will require your body to burn several pounds of fat a week as a source of energy. Doing lots of sit ups and leg raises will not reduce your percentage of body fat.

IS IT IMPOSSIBLE TO SPOT REDUCE?

Yes! On a reducing diet, fat is mobilized out of the multiple fat cells all over you body, then carried by the bloodstream to the individual active cells in your body, and burned for energy. Thus, fat stores are withdrawn from your total body fat cells and not from one isolated location. Individual exercises will develop your muscles but they will do little or nothing to reduce your percentage of body fat.

DON'T ANY SPOT-REDUCING GADGETS WORK?

No! Not only do they not result in permanent fat loss, but many of these gadgets are dangerous. Let us examine some of the most popular ones:

1. Motorized exercycles— An exercycle is a motorized bicycle that moves your legs and torso for you. Since the machine is pulling your legs up and down, it is doing the work, not you.

2. Electrical shock— This machine supposedly makes the muscles contract involuntarily through small electric charges. Actually, the muscle movements are too small to consume enough energy to cause a noticeable reduction in fat. Doctors believe certain of these machines can be dangerous to the heart and other organs which respond to the electric stimuli.

3. Vibrating belts—A mechanical vibrating belt may relax you and make you feel better, but it certainly will not remove fat. Fat cannot be shaken, tickled, beaten, or stroked from your body.

4. Rubber clothes— These clothes, which range from belts, shorts, and shirts to full outfits, are supposed to make you "sweat off" the fat and inches. Any weight you lose this way is simply the result of dehydration, which is quickly eradicated when you quench your thirst. None of the water you lose when you sweat comes from your body fat, since fat contains just a small percentage of water.

5. Sauna wraps— In this principle, your body (or the specific part you want reduced) is wrapped with tape, which has been soaked

in a "secret" solution. You then sit in a sauna bath for thirty minutes, and--supposedly--the secret solution draws the excess fat from your body. Again, you CANNOT passively sweat fat off your body.

HOW CAN I BUILD UP MY "WIND"?

Three factors are important in developing cardiorespiratory endurance or "wind." First, exercise must be of sufficient intensity to increase the heart rate to at least one hundred forty beats per minute. Second, this heart rate must be sustained for at least ten to twelve minutes. Third, the exercise bout should be repeated three to four times a week.

In general, the more the body's large musculature involved in the exercise, the easier it will be for your heart rate to exceed one hundred forty beats per minute. For example, bicycling, jogging, swimming, and proper weight training are much better cardiorespiratory exercises that an equal amount of softball, golf, or tennis.

IS THERE ANY DIFFERENCE BETWEEN MUSCULAR SIZE AND STRENGTH?

Everything else being equal, a big muscle is a strong muscle. In other words, there is a close relationship between the size of a muscle and its strength. Increase one of the factors, and the other also increases.

Some confusion, however, occurs in the phrase: "everything else being equal." That is why you occasionally see a man with large muscles who cannot demonstrate strength as well as a man with smaller muscles; "everything else" is usually not equal.

Ability to lift a barbell (demonstrating strength) is composed of many factors. For example, bodily proportion (leverage), neurological efficiency, and skill at lifting a barbell are also important. This is why it is almost impossible to compare the muscular strength of one individual to the strength of another. Too many factors are involved.

The best thing to do is to compare you with yourself. By keeping accurate records over a period of time, you will know if you are getting stronger, your muscles are also increasing in size.

WHAT DETERMINES MY MUSCULAR POTENTIAL?

Your muscular potential is primarily determined by the length of your muscles. Not the length of the bone, but the length of the muscle (contractile tissue) from where the tendon attaches to the muscle at one end to where the tendon attaches to the same muscle at the other end. Muscle lengths or bellies that can easily be measured are triceps of the arm, gastrocnemius of the calf, and flexors of the forearm.

If two men flex the long head of the triceps (with the arm down by the side) and you measured the length of this muscle, you might find vastly different measurements. For example, the length of the first man's triceps might measure six inches while the second man's measures nine inches. The length of the second man's triceps is 50% longer than the first man's triceps. As a result the second man has the potential to have 2.25 times as much cross sectional area (1.5 X 1.5=2.25) and 3.375 as much volumn or mass (1.5 X 1.5 X 1.5=3.375) to his triceps. Untrained, both of these men may have approximately the same size arm; but, with proper training, the second man can have a much stronger and larger triceps muscle.

Thus, the length of a given muscle determines its ultimate size. The length of a man's muscles is genetic in nature and not subject to improvement.

WHICH TYPE OF EQUIPMENT CAN MAKE ME STRONGEST?

As I said before, one requirement for developing muscular size and strength is high-intensity exercise. You can use the high-intensity principle with most types of equipment. However, for maximum size and strength increases in the shortest possible time, you must use equipment that provides full-range exercise.

A word of explanation is needed about full-range exercise. An exercise is full-range only if it provides resistance throughout the entire movement of the involved body parts. Resistance must be provided in the extended (starting) position, throughout the mid-range, and in the contracted (finishing) position. Exercise equipment which lacks any of these three basic requirements is not full range.

Barbells, Universal, Isokinetics, and Nautilus all provide resistance in the mid-range of movement, but only the Nautilus provides resistance in both the starting and finishing positions. On the other hand, barbells and Universal can provide resistance in either the starting or finishing position (depending on the exercise), but never in both. Isokinetic exercises have no resistance in either of these two positions.

Nautilus machines are also superior because they provide rotary movement, direct resistance, variable resistance, and balanced resistance. Therefore, if you have access to Nautilus equipment, be sure and take advantage of it. You will definitely get faster and better results.

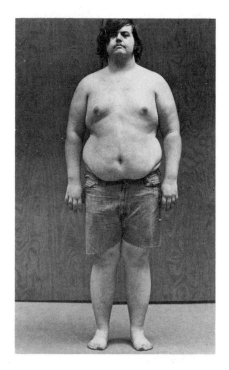

Photo 1 shows Sammie Johns on the first of January when he weighed 299 pounds. Twenty-three year old Mr. Johns then began a physical fitness program under the supervision of the author. Prior to this time, he ate one meal a day, a continuous one that began after he finished work at 5:30 P.M. and continued until he went to bed about 11:00 P.M. His only recreational activity was twisting on the TV knobs and bending to get beer and cheese out of the refrigerator.

Photo 2 shows Sammie Johns six months later. On the first of July he weighed only 182 pounds. That is a reduction of 117 pounds of fat! During his individualized fitness program, Mr. Johns was encouraged to eat three small meals a day. He was also motivated to exercise vigorously every other day.

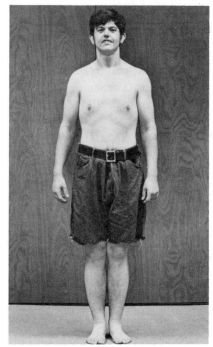

WHICH EXERCISES WILL HELP ME IN FOOTBALL?

For football, or for any sport, you must decide which muscle groups should be developed and which ones should not. Football happens to be a sport which requires greater than average strength in all major muscle groups. Basketball, tennis, and baseball players also require overall strength, while golfers, swimmers, and gymnasts need to concentrate more on their upper body development.

If the Nautilus equipment is available, I recommend using the following machines:

Hip and Back	Leg Extension
Leg Press	Leg Curl
Pullover	Double Shoulder
Neck and Shoulder	Double Chest
Biceps/Triceps	4-Way Neck
Rotary Neck	

The following conventional exercises may be substituted if the Nautilus machines are not available:

Squat(barbell)	Standing curl(barbell)
Leg press(leg press machine)	Dip(parallel bars)
Stiff-legged deadlift (barbell)	Neck harness
Shoulder shrug (barbell, dumbells)	Standing press (barbell)
Chin-up, palms-up grip	Bench press(barbell)
(horizontal bar)	
Bent-armed Pullover(barbell or dumbbells)	

HOW OFTEN SHOULD I TRAIN?

In an earlier question, I pointed out that many trainees confuse "intensity of training" with a "large amount of training." If you train in a high intensity fashion, you cannot stand much exercise. This means that if you are a beginning trainee, you should exercise every other day (three times a week--Monday, Wednesday, Friday). You should perform one set of each exercise, and it should take you no more than forty minutes, at the most, to complete the routine. Advanced trainees, because they can handle much heavier resistance with more intensity, must train even less----only two times a week. Remember, brief workouts two or three times a week are best.

82

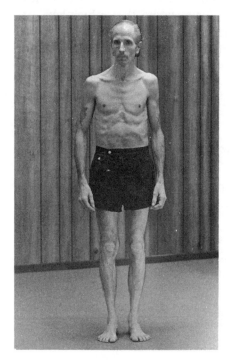

When this photo was taken, Lewis Thursby was forty-two years old, and weighed a mere 104 pounds even though he was 5 feet 8 inches tall. He was actually "under fat, " as well as being "under muscled" at his body weight.

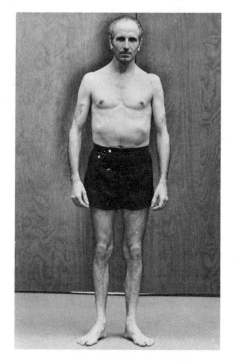

After three months of supervised exercise and nutrition, Mr. Thursby weighed 142 pounds, an increase of 38 pounds. He also doubled his strength. During this three-month period, he ate five medium-sized meals a day and exercised on Nautilus equipment three times a week.

WHAT ABOUT STRENGTH TRAINING DURING THE SEASON?

Many players make the mistake of progressing in their strength training until the season starts, and then they slack off or totally ignor training afterward. As a result, their strength level decreases with each missed workout. In fact, studies have shown that a high level of strength development shows measureable degeneration after as little as ninety-six hours of normal activity. Therefore, to maintain or increase muscular strength during the season, you should continue your high-intensity training at least twice a week. If possible, workouts should be performed the day after the game and then again three days later.

DO SOME ATHLETES TAKE HORMONE DRUGS TO DEVELOP LARGER MUSCLES?

Yes, some take a drug that is the synthtic derivative of the male hormone testosterone. It is prescribed and sold under the brand names of Dianabol, Anavar, Nilevar, and Winstrol. Athletes, coaches, and even some medical people have assumed that if a certain amount of male hormone is responsible for muscular development, then adding more to this already adequate chemical balance will produce a stimulus for larger muscles. This is simply not true.

More is not better when it comes to your hormone balance. These drugs do have a place for patients with burns, glandular inbalances, etc.; but, at no time will a healthy athlete benefit physiologically from them.

The trouble with the whole drug scene is that athletes, because they are some of the world's worst faddists may "think" (placebo effect) they are getting stronger faster from a certain pill. As a result, they continue to take them in larger doses and more frequently (the old "more is better" syndrome). Eventually, if such drugging continues for a long time, the body may lose its ability to produce such hormones naturally; and a man could be turned into a eunuch.

DO PROTEIN SUPPLEMENTS AND VITAMIN PILLS HELP?

You do need to have a certain amount of protein and various vitamins present in your body to carry forth with the muscular growth processes once they have started. But, if you eat a balanced diet composed of a variety of foods, you are certain to get more than enough of the various nutrients for maximum muscular growth.

To simplify matters, nutritionists have divided foods into four basic groups:(1) Meat, (2) Dairy, (3)Fruit and Vegetable, (4) Bread and Cereal. For a well-balanced diet, nutritionists recommend at least one serving from each of the four food groups at each meal. Generally speaking, if you adhere to these guidelines, you will not need to waste your money on protein supplements and vitamin pills.

In the final analysis, your training programs should be designed with two goals in mind: (1) the production of maximum strength of the muscles involved on your sport, and (2) the reduction or elimination of body fat to a minimum. Both of these goals can be accomplished through high-intensity exercise along with a reasonable diet.

PART
B

FITNESS-RELATED
TOPICS

INTRODUCTION TO FITNESS-RELATED TOPICS

Dissatisfied with your physical fitness? Article nine describes a simple test that you can take to evaluate your strength, flexibility, and heart-lung efficiency. It also contains some helpful hints on how to improve you fitness.

Some women are currently involved in jogging; and many more would be interested if they knew how to jog, how much, and how often. Article ten lists some easy to understand guidelines for you to follow. In addition, " How to Outrun the Gingerbread Man" is a roundabout way of telling you how to avoid some of the pitfalls and problems associated with jogging.

"The Swim for Lunch Bunch" is a story about a group of fitness-minded people at Florida State University who gear their lunch hour around the swimming pool. Beginning, intermediate, and advanced guidlelines are suggested for those of you who would like to swim your way to fitness.

Have you noticed the large number of people who are riding bicycles to and from work---or, for fitness and fun? Why not join in the good times? There is a bicycle built that is just right for you. Of course, the "how to's" and important guidelines are in this article, too.

You will probably have some unanswered questions by this point in the book. Thirteen, "Misconceptions About Exercise ," picks up the pieces and fills in the gaps left by the preceding articles.

"How to Get in Shape for Pregnancy," the subject for article fourteen, attempts to separate myth and supersition from facts. After reading the article, you should see the value of progressive resistance exercise during and after pregnancy.

Tired, lacking in energy, and don't know why? Then, don't skip article fifteen. It's written just for you. The article is about fatigue. What is it? How do you recognize it? And, more importantly, what do you do about it? These questions and more are answered.

Article sixteen wraps up Part B by giving some useful hints on "how to relax" in just five short minutes. You'll want to read this article several times.

How Fit
Are You?
A Simple Test

9

HOW FIT ARE YOU? A SIMPLE TEST

Let's assume you accidentally drop this book on the floor. You reach down to get it. As you straighten up, the weak muscles in your back stretch----pull----and finally tear.

In pain and fear you grab your back and with the other hand you reach for support. This action causes you to twist your body. Once again you feel a sharp pain----this time in the lower back.

Fear and pain cause your heart to beat wildly----faster and faster. Suddenly, it feels like an anvil has been dropped on your chest. Pain pounds your breastbone and radiates down your left arm. You gasp for air!

In less than a minute, you have wrenched a back muscle, slipped a disc, and had a heart attack. You ARE in bad shape, because you WERE in bad shape.

"It can't happen to me," you say.

Can't it? An estimated 100 million people in the United States are overweight and out-of-shape. These people are prime candidates for pulled muscles, slipped discs, and heart attacks. Are you one of them?

Most of you know you are in bad shape, and you earnestly wish you were in better shape. One problem you must face, though, are all the misconceptions, false beliefs, and outright lies that surround the world of physical fitness and exercise. Unless you are an expert, it is really hard to determine what kind of exercise and how much is best for you.

Therefore, the purpose of this article is to give you positive guidelines for getting in shape and staying there.

Let's begin by defining physical fitness.

WHAT IS PHYSICAL FITNESS?

Physical fitness is defined as your ability to work vigorously, without undue fatigue, with energy left for enjoying recreational activities and for meeting unforeseen emergencies.

Think about that definition for a minute. Can you meet the demands of your life? If someone asked you to go ice skating this evening, would you eagerly accept? Or would you be too tired, or afraid you might pull a muscle or slip a disc? Perhaps with that bulging waistline and fat hips you fear you might make a spectacle of yourself?

How about the other demands of life. Could you respond to an emergency by carrying someone out of a burning house? Could you defend yourself against a mugger?

To be able to follow through in your work with vigor and pleasure and still have something left over, you must understand all the factors that make up physical fitness. Awareness and understanding of these factors will go a long way toward getting you in shape.

COMPONENTS OF PHYSICAL FITNESS

The success of your program is based on the measurement, evaluation, and improvement of the four components of physical fitness: muscular strength, flexibility, heart-lung efficiency, and body fat. While there are many ways of measuring and evaluating these factors, for practical purposes, you can get an idea of your present condition by taking the following tests.

Muscular Strength. Muscular strength, or the ability to exert force against resistance, is determined by your performance in the chin-up (arm hang for women) and squat thrust.

Chin-up (for arm and shoulder strength). Men, hang from a bar with your palms facing you and pull until your chin is over the bar. Your legs must hang without kicking. Lower to a straight arm position. Count the number of times your chin goes over the bar. Women, hang from the bar with your arms straight and feet off the floor for as long as possible. Record your hanging time in seconds.

Squat-thrust (for leg and back strength). Stand, then bend your knees and place your hands on the floor in front of your feet. Thrust your legs back far enough so that your body is perfectly straight from shoulders to feet. Return to the squat position. Then return to the standing position. Practice until you learn the movement, and then count the number of squat thrusts you can do in ten seconds.

Flexibility. Flexibility is the range of movement of a body segment around the joint. It is measured by the toe touch and back raise.

Toe Touch (lower back and leg flexibility). Keeping your legs together and knees locked, bend at the waist and try to touch the floor with your fingertips. Women should try to touch the floor with their palms.

Back Raise (upper and lower back flexibility). Lying flat on your stomach, with your fingers laced behind your neck and your feet pinned to the floor, raise your chin and chest as far as possible. Hold steady until a friend can measure the vertical distance from the floor to your chin.

91

How Fit Are You? A Simple Test

Heart-Lung Efficiency. This is the ability of the circulatory and respiratory systems to support activities that require sustained effort. This efficiency is tested by running in place.

Running in place. Run in place for sixty seconds, lifting your feet at least four inches from the floor. Then take three deep breaths, and hold the last one for as many seconds as you can without breathing.

Body Fat Analysis. Body fat is the excess fat that is stored under your skin. It is measured by the "pinch test."

"Pinch test." At least 50% of your body fat is deposited directly under the skin. The thickness of the skin and its underlying fat can be measured with special tension calipers or with the fingers. Pick up a pinch of the skin from the back of the arm, midway between the elbow and shoulder (mid-triceps area). When you take your fingers away, have a ruler handy so that you can measure the distance between your fingers (to the nearest eighth of an inch). Research has shown that the thickness of the skin in the mid-triceps area correlates fairly well to the total body fat determined by comprehensive measurements. In addition, research shows that the average American has twice as much fat under his skin as he needs for optimum fitness.

You can quickly evaluate your performance on the six tests by looking at the table below. The table lists only minimum performances. Anything below these standards means that you are more susceptible to the vast array of physical deterioration diseases that exist.

PHYSICAL FITNESS SCORING TABLE

Components	Minimum or Passing Scores MEN	WOMEN
1. Muscular Strength		
Pull-ups	3	30 second hang
Squat thrusts	4 in 10 seconds	3 in 10 seconds
2. Flexibility		
Toe touch	fingertips on floor	palms on floor
Back raise	18 inches or more from chin to floor	16 inches or more from chin to floor

92

3. **Heart-Lung Efficiency**
   Holding breath after run-
   ning in place   30 seconds   25 seconds
4. **Body Fat**
   "Pinch test"   1/2 inch   3/4 inch
                                    or less   or less

Now that you have an evaluation of your present physical condition, I am going to tell you what to do about your weak points. However, before involving yourself in this program, you can do your part by getting your doctor's approval. If possible, you should have a thorough medical examination that includes a cardiological stress-test.

IMPROVING YOUR PHYSICAL FITNESS

Muscular Strength. Careful research by Dr. Paavo Komi of Finland has shown that for building muscular strength, lowering resistance (negative work) is far more effective than raising resistance (positive work). Why? For several reasons: one, you can always lower a heavier weight than you can raise, thus the intensity of the exercise can be higher; two, lowering a weight produces less intramuscular friction than raising a weight. In some respects, this makes smaller inroads into your overall recovery ability.

How can the concept of lowering resistance or negative work be used to help you improve your strength? First, try to think of ways you can accentuate the lowering portion of traditional exercise. For example, let us take the chin-up, push-up, deep-knee bend, and sit-up.

In the chin-up, you use your legs to help you get your chin over the bar. Simply place a wooden box in front of the horizontal bar and step up on the box (rather than pulling up with your arms) until your chin is over the bar. Lower yourself very slowly (6 to 8 seconds). Climb back and repeat.

Push-ups can be performed in a similar manner by simply using your knees and lower back to help you straighten your arms. Then you should lower yourself slowly (again 6 to 8 seconds) until your chest touches the floor.

For stomach conditioning and strength, you will want to try the negative-accentuated sit-up. With your knees slightly bent, feet securely held down, hands behind head, slowly lower your upper body until your back touches the floor. Once on the floor, use your arms to assist you in sitting up.

The deep knee bend can be done in several different fashions. You can bend your legs very slowly (you may want to work up to 10 to 15 seconds lowering on this one), and quickly stand up and repeat. Or, you can lower yourself with one leg (you may need a chair to hold on to for balance), stand up on two legs, and lower yourself on the opposite leg.

For best results from these movements, try to perform one set of eight to twelve repetitions, three times a week.

Also, if you give the concept some additional thought, I am sure you will see ways you can apply the negative accentuated style of training to barbells and weight machines.

Flexibility. Dr. James A. Peterson of the United States Military Academy at West Point, New York, has found that three factors are important in building heart-lung efficiency. One, the exercise must be hard enough to get your heart rate up to 140-150 beats a minute. Two, then you must sustain this heart rate for ten to twelve minutes. Three, such exercise should be repeated three times a week.

At first, you may be able to sustain a heart rate of 140 beats a minute for only two or three minutes. If this is the case, then you will need to improve your efficiency in each of these three areas.

In general, the more of a body's musculature involved in exercise, the easier it will be to reach a heart rate of 140-150 beats a minute. Bicycling, swimming, jogging, running-in-place, and even fast walking are good examples of large muscle exercises.

Learn to take your own heart rate (or pulse rate) during and after exercise by counting the beats for ten seconds and multiplying by six to get the beats per minute.

For best results, you should work on improving your strength, flexibility, and heart-lung efficiency all the same day with a day of rest in between. In other words, an every-other-day program is best.

How to Outrun
the Gingerbread Man

10

HOW TO OUTRUN THE GINGERBREAD MAN

Run, run as fast as you can,
You can't catch me,
I'm the Gingerbread Man.

Remember the story about the Gingerbread Man?

The Gingerbread Man was running to get his freedom. He didn't just want to exist inside the cookie box—-waiting to be eaten by some hungry person. No! He wanted to be involved in life as an active participant. Therefore, when the door opened, he made his move and into the great outdoors he ran.

Have you ever felt like the Gingerbread Man? Boxed up all day, behind a desk or in front of an oven, just existing?

Now's the time for you to do something about this feeling. Open the door, get outside, and run, run, run!

Authorities agree that running is one of the best ways to become physically fit. Many state and local heart associations have started "Run For Your Life" programs in communities across the nation. Physicians support running as an excellent cardiovascular exercise. Popular magazines have printed numerous reports on the improvement in physical fitness due to running. Last year over 2,000 people entered the Boston Marathon. The age of the majority of entrants was over twenty-six. In addition, it is estimated that some five million people in the United States are presently involved in running or jogging programs.

Considerable research indicates that people participating in a running program may increase their cardiovascular fitness to such a level that the risk of coronary disease is lessened. Regular physical activity has also been shown to reduce serum cholesterol and triglyceride level, high blood pressure, and body fat. Also, running is recommended by many pyschiatrists as a means of relieving tension and stress of everyday living.

When you consider any exercise program, especially running, there are some important facts you should know. There are many advantages to running, but there are also some dangers you should be aware of. It can be very dangerous to those who have joint and lower back problems. Here, though, are some of the advantages:

ADVANTAGES OF RUNNING

It is free. Not a thing about running costs you a cent. You may have to expend a little will power to start, but that should not bankrupt you.

How to Outrun the Gingerbread Man

No special equipment. Many fitness programs cost a great deal before the first workout. This is not so with running. Other than proper shoes, your body is the only equipment necessary.

No special facilities. No gymnasium, tennis courts, or pools. Just open the door and you are in business.

It is quick. There are 1,440 minutes in a day. Initially running takes about thirty minutes, three times a week, or ninety minutes out of 10,080 minutes a week. That is not much time to devote to fitness. If you are not willing to spend this minimum time for better fitness, you had better be prepared to spend even more of it being sick.

Old and young can do it. Anyone from nine to ninety who is not sick or disabled can benefit from a graduated program of running. Thousands of runners are proving this every day.

Improves you heart and lungs. A graduated running program does much to improve the heart, lungs, and circulatory system by progressively expanding your capacity to handle stress.

You feel and look better. Running stimulates circulation, tones the muscles, and produces a more optimistic outlook. It reduces the hips and thighs, firms sagging muscles, and flattens the abdomen. Also, those who are in good condition are more active sexually. There is a psychological element as well. If you look and feel better, you gain confidence. Because you feel more attractive, you are more attractive.

Helps you lose fat. A good program of running can reduce the amount of fat on your body and at the same time increase the amount of muscle. Running, along with a careful diet, guarantees a desirable fat loss.

Builds endurance and confidence. Running makes you more fit. You can confidently tackle your job, increase your work load, or set out to enjoy a recreational activity without fear of overexerting your heart.

Smaller waistline. Running helps to redistribute weight. In controlled programs, nearly all runners reduced the size of their waistline. In addition, women joggers dropped a dress size.

Run alone or with others. If you crave time alone, then run by yourself. You can think without distraction or just put your mind to sleep. On the other hand, if you like company, group running provides great companionship.

How to Outrun the Gingerbread Man

PRECAUTIONS AND PREPARATIONS

A running program, whether it be for middle-aged adults, youngsters, or oldsters, should have some built-in precautions.

One of the first precautions is get your physician's approval. This is especially important for the "over thirty" and "over forty" age group. Most people can follow a running training schedule with little difficulty other than the normal aches and pains. But, there are exceptions. **Play it safe and get a complete medical examination.** If possible, this should include a cardiological stress-test.

If you have spent more than twenty years getting out of shape, do not expect to see immediate results. Try to realize that there is a preliminary period during which you should become conditioned to moderate exercise before any strenuous exercise is undertaken. The older you are, the longer the preparation period should be. The correct way to begin any fitness program is to start slowly and progress at a steady but slow rate.

Some people choose to run out of doors on highways and sidewalks. Since the surfaces they run on are hard and non-resilient, they put stress on the heels and legs that can cause soreness. Therefore, the best place to run is a grassy area. A grassy turf has some spring and give in it. That makes it easier on your ankles and knee joints. Where no grassy area is handy, any surface will do provided you wear the proper shoes---ones with sturdy absorbent soles and a good cushion inside that will provide an artifical softness.

You will need to know how far you are running. For example, are you running 100 yards, 1/4 mile, or more? This can easily be calculated on your local high school track. Each straight away and each turn is 110 yards. Once around the track is 1/4 mile or 440 yards, and four times around the track equals one mile.

If no track is available, you can map out your course around the neighborhood by measuring the distance on your car's odometer. Use the tenth of a mile figure in the right hand column. Or, you can always walk off a course yourself. The average stride is about one yard.

Prior to running, you should warm-up by doing a few calisthenic exercises. These should consist of arm circling, twisting the trunk side to side while standing, toe touching, and standing with your feet widely apart and stretching the inside of your thighs by bending your left leg and then your right leg.

PRIMARY RUNNING MUSCLES AND THEIR ACTIONS

At first glance the running motion itself may seem quite easy. However, it is a very complex movement that involves many muscles. The primary running muscles are divided into six groups. As you read this section, please refer to the drawing for a better understanding of the muscles involved.

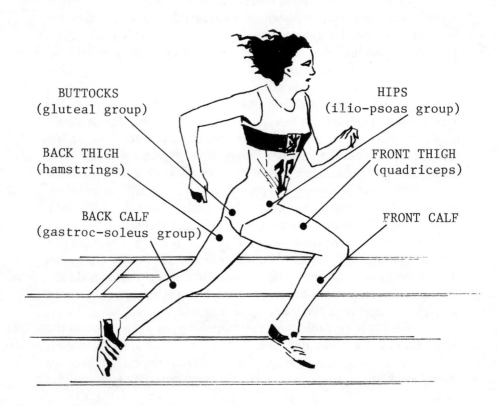

BUTTOCKS
(gluteal group)

HIPS
(ilio-psoas group)

BACK THIGH
(hamstrings)

FRONT THIGH
(quadriceps)

BACK CALF
(gastroc-soleus group)

FRONT CALF

How to Outrun the Gingerbread Man

1. Buttocks (gluteal group). This large and powerful muscle group extends from the hip bone (pelvis) to the lower spinal column to the fascia of the upper thigh. The primary function of the buttocks is to thrust the thigh backward, thus propelling the trunk forward. Your power stroke in running comes from your buttock muscles. In fact, the faster you run, the more dependent upon your buttocks you become. The next time you are at a track meet or football game, notice that all great sprinters, hurdlers, jumpers, fullbacks, and halfbacks have large, well-developed buttocks.

2. Hips (ilio-psoas group). These muscles originate at the lower spinal column and pelvis and are inserted into the upper thigh bone. In running, they move the thigh forward.

3. Back thigh (hamstrings) These muscles extend from the pelvis and upper thigh to the bones of the calf (tibia and fibula). The primary action of the hamstrings is to force the calf backward.

4. Front thigh (quadriceps). Four strong muscles make up the quadriceps. They extend from the hip and upper thigh to the kneecap. Straightening the knee, thus thrusting the leg forward, is their major function.

5. Back calf. This is composed of two muscles that extend from the lower thigh and upper tibia and fibula to the heel bone by way of the leg tendon (Achilles). Their function in running is to spring the foot off the ground.

6. Front calf. These muscles extend from the upper calf to the ones of the foot. They raise the ball of the foot.

HOW TO RUN

One of the mistakes commonly made by leaders of fitness programs is to assume that everyone knows how to run. Unfortunately, this is not the case. Let us look at the techniques and movements involved in efficient running.

1. Body inclined slightly forward at the ankles, degree increasing with speed.

2. Free leg swings from hips, movement line straight forward and backward.

3. Emphasis on knee-lift forward with limited pickup behind.

4. Landing on heel, then ball of foot, and toes in slow running; on ball of foot and toes in sprinting.

5. Forceful pushoff with toes.

6. Knee are stabilized if a conscious effort is made to run slightly pigeon-toed.

7. Abdominal muscles firm to stabilize trunk and mobilize force.

8. Spring with ankle and foot.

9. Elbows bent at right angles, arms close to sides and swinging in opposition to legs.

10. Dangle arms and hands occasionally.

11. Chin and chest high.

12. Breathe with your mouth open.

TRAINING PRINCIPLES

Study these training principles and keep them in mind as you begin your running program.

Train, don't strain. This is the golden rule of running. Although it is not harmful to go all out once you are in good condition, this should be attempted only occasionally.

Gradual stress. Moderation underlies the principle of gradually increasing stress. The runner who can run the mile in six minutes does not prepare for a five minute mile by trying to run one every day. A better way is to advance toward a goal a little bit each day, each week, each month, by making use of sound physiological facts. Running is a gradual, moderate exercise that permits you to tone your body while working within your own capability. The gradual stress prevents over exertion and the danger of an unaccustomed burden on the heart, lungs, and other parts of the body.

Variety. Exercise should be interesting. The same exercises done in the same place, at the same time, every day can bring on indifference. Therefore, it is important to include as much variety as possible in your program. You can run almost anywhere----in the country, in the park, at the beach, in a vacant lot, and even in your home or office. It is important for you to lay out your schedule with ample variety.

Plan. You should work by plan because order is helpful. Expert runners know what they are going to do each day for a month or even months in advance. Yet, the plan is not rigid. It can be modified at any time. Working by a plan helps increase moderation, variety, and regularity.

Regularity. The benefits of running will vary directly with your regularity in following your program. Obviously, one week on and one week off will not produce the results that regular exercise will. There are no lasting benefits to health when you exercise a short time and stop. You should strive to run three to five times a week. Some people make good progress by running every other day, others like a five-times-a-week schedule. Anything below two times a week is almost useless and probably harmful.

Pace and Duration. Once you get accustomed to running, two factors, pace and duration, are important to producing a desired training effect. By training effect, I am referring to stimulating the heart and making it beat more efficiently. Exercising for the average person under thirty should be strenuous enough to produce a heart rate of at least 150 beats per minute. This can be determined by finding the pulse at your wrist or neck and counting the beats for ten seconds. You can do this during or immediately after exercise and multiply by six for an estimate of the pace of the exercise. A heart rate of 150 beats per minute means that you are working at about 60% of your maximum capacity. That is a good energy level for producing a training effect in young, healthy people.

The training effect, however, can be produced in other ways. For example, you may work for a short time at a high heart rate or a longer time at a slower heart rate. The following chart shows some combinations which can be used in achieving the training effect.

Training Effect

Daily Time Requirements (Min.)	*90*	*45*	*20*	*10*
Working Capacity (% of Max.)	*30*	*40*	*50*	*60*
Heart Rate (beats per min.)	*120*	*130*	*140*	*150*

The longer periods are more realistic for older people, whereas the exercises for younger people can be harder and shorter.

A SUGGESTED TRAINING SCHEDULE

This training schedule is designed and suggested for inexperienced and/or out-of-condition runners. To determine your condition, you can take the 12-minute run-walk test that was developed by Dr. Kenneth H. Cooper. All you need for this test is a measured track and a watch with a second hand. Try to run or walk as fast as you can in twelve minutes. If you cannot cover at least .85 to 1 mile or 3.5 to 4 laps, you are in VERY POOR condition. If you can cover more than a mile, you will probably need to start on a harder program.

In the following program, the progress should be relatively slow, depending on the age and condition of the runner. Remember, too, that although this is primarily a running program, it is also important to strengthen the muscles of the abdomen, shoulder girdle, and back. You should, therefore, include three or four calisthenic-type exercises in your daily workouts. Better yet, incorporate a strength-training routine within your program.

First Week *(every other day or three times per week)*

1. Warm-up with stretching, twisting and bending exercises. Concentrate on the muscles in the back of your legs and insides of the thighs.

2. Walk 200 yards.

3. Touch your toes, stretch your legs, twist at the waist, and circle your arms.

4. Jog approximately 50 yards, walk 50 yards (6 times).

5. Jog approximately 100 yards, walk 100 yards (3 times).

6. Cool down by walking approximately 200 yards.

Second Week

1,2,3 as in First Week.

4. Jog 50 yards, walk 50 yards (8 times).

5. Jog 100 yards, walk 100 yards (4 times).

6. Cool down by walking 200 yards.

At the end of the second week your muscles should begin to adapt to the exercise. The intermediate running program may be started at this time. The following is suggested as a four week schedule from the third to the sixth week.

Third Week

1. Warm up.

2. Run 100 yards, walk 100 yards (8 times).

3. Rest 3 minutes.

4. Jog 300 yards.

5. Walk 200 yards to cool down.

Fourth Week

1. Warm-up.

2. Run 100 yards, walk 100 yards (10 times).

3. Rest 3 minutes.

4. *Jog 600 yards.*
5. *Walk 200 yards to cool down.*

Fifth Week

1. *Warm-up.*
2. *Run 150 yards, walk 100 yards (8 times).*
3. *Rest 3 minutes.*
4. *Run 600 yards.*
5. *Walk 200 yards to cool down.*

Sixth Week

1. *Warm-up.*
2. *Run 200 yards, walk 100 yards (8 times).*
3. *Rest 3 minutes.*
4. *Run 880 yards or 1/2 mile.*
5. *Walk 400 yards to cool down.*

After this six-week program, you should again test yourself on the 12-minute run-walk test. You should now be able to jog continuously for the entire twelve minutes. Hopefully you will be able to cover five or six laps or 1 1/4 to 1 1/2 miles. Also, your heart rate should be around 140 beats a minute for most of the twelve minutes.

From this point on, you should be able to devise your own schedule by increasing your running distance and speed. Be sure that warm-up and cool-down always precede and follow the workout.

If you are under thirty-five, let the following distances, times, and frequencies serve as a goal to strive toward. When you can consistantly perform any one of these programs, you can be certain you have obtained a high degree of fitness.

FINAL GOAL

DISTANCE (MILES)	TIME (MIN.) REQUIREMENT	FREQUENCY WEEK
1.0	8:15	4
1.5	14:00	4
1.5	12:30	3
2.0	20:15	3
2.0	16:30	2

How to Outrun the Gingerbread Man

WARNINGS

After starting your jogging program, certain situations may occur that indicate you are doing too much. The warnings listed in the table are not meant to frighten you, but they are meant to provide you with an understanding of the minor aches and pains associated with a beginning exercise program.

While some warnings may occur during an exercise session, it is important to know that certain symptoms may also occur some two to twenty-four hours later. The table distinguishes between immediate and delayed symptoms.

The first three symptoms are cause for consulting a physician. If you cannot get in touch with him, discontinue your jogging program. Symptoms four through eight have suggested remedies that may be tried prior to consulting a physician.

The other symptoms can usually be remedied without medical advise by the measures described. However, if the suggested measures fail to work, prompt medical help should be sought.

CONCLUSION

Oh, yes, you are probably still wondering about the Gingerbread Man.

Well, the Gingerbread Man so the story goes, outran the old woman, the old man, the bunny rabbit, and the bear cub. But he met his match with the sly fox.

No, the fox did not chase the Gingerbread Man down. He outsmarted the Gingerbread Man by persuading him to go across the river on his back. As a result, half-way across the river he became a tasty meal for the sly fox.

If the Gingerbread Man had used his head as well as his legs, he would probably still be running today.

Thus, the moral of this story is: Not only must you be motivated to exercise and run, but you should know how to organize a sound training progam and proceed with it in a sensible manner.

---SO----

Run, run as fast as you can,
But be more cautious
Than the Gingerbread Man!

Warnings and What to Do About Them

Symptom	Cause	Remedy
1. Abnormal heart rate; e.g. pulse becoming irregular; fluttering, jumping, or palpitations in chest or throat; sudden burst of rapid heartbeats; sudden very slow pulse. (immediate or delayed)	Extrasystoles (extra heart beats), dropped heartbeats, or disorders of cardiac rhythm. May or may not be dangerous.	Consult physician before resuming exercise program. May be a completely harmless kind of cardiac rhythm disorder.
2. Pain or pressure in the center of the chest or the arm or throat precipitated by exercise or following exercise. (immediate or delayed)	Possible heart problem.	Consult physician before resuming exercise program.
3. Dizziness, lightheadedness, confusion, cold sweat, glassy stare, pallor, blueness or fainting. (immediate)	Insufficient blood to the brain.	Do not try to cool down. Stop exercise and lie down with feet elevated, or put head down between legs until symptoms pass. Later consult physician before next exercise session.
4. Persistent rapid heart rate 5-10 minutes after the exercise was stopped. (immediate)	Exercise is probably too vigorous.	Increase the vigor of exercise more slowly. If these measures do not control the excessively high recovery rate, consult physician.
5. Flare-up of arthritic condition or gout which usually occurs in hips, knees, ankles, or big toe. (immediate or delayed)	Trauma to joints which are particularly vulnerable.	If you are familiar with how to quiet these flare-ups of your old joint condition, use usual remedies. Rest and do not resume exercise program until condition subsides. Then resume the exercise at a lower level with protective footwear on softer surfaces.
6. Pain around the knee. (delayed)	Usually related to the kneecap (patella) if it is not firmly fixed in large tendon in which it is contained. If the kneecap isn't centered firmly and properly in the tendon, increased wear and friction result.	Strengthen muscles that surround the knee: the quadriceps and hamstrings. Practice jogging in a slightly pigeon-toed fashion using shoes with thicker soles.
7. Soreness in the tendon (Achilles) that connects the calf to the heel bone. (delayed)	Lack of flexibility in large calf muscles (gastrocnemius).	Work on progressively stretching the calf muscles by standing off a ledge on the balls of your feet and gently lowering your heels.
8. Foot pain, especially in the ball. (immediate and delayed)	Improperly fitted shoes and faulty running technique.	Firm arch and heel support, thick resilient soles to absorb the impact. When running, practice landing on your heels. If symptoms persist, see a podiatrist.

How to Outrun the Gingerbread Man

Symptom	Cause	Remedy
9. Nausea or vomiting after exercise. (immediate)	Not enough oxygen to the intestine. You are either exercising too vigorously or cooling off too quickly.	Exercise less vigorously and be sure to take a more gradual and longer cool-down.
10. Prolonged fatigue even 24 hours delayed. (delayed)	Exercise is too vigorous.	Increase your level more gradually.
11. Shin splints (pain on the front or sides of calf). (delayed)	Inflammation of the fascia connecting the leg bones, or muscle tears where muscles of the lower leg connect to the bones.	Use shoes with thicker soles. Jog on turf which is easier on your legs. Strengthen your front calf muscles.
12. Insomnia which was not present prior to the exercise program. (delayed)	Exercise is too vigorous.	Reduce exercise to lower level, then increase intensity of exercise gradually.
13. Pain in the calf muscles which occurs on heavy exercise but not at rest. (immediate)	May be due to muscle cramps from lack of use of these muscles, or exercising on hard surfaces.	Use shoes with thicker soles, cool down adequately. Muscle cramps should clear up after a few sessions.
14. Side stitch (aching under the ribs while jogging). (immediate)	Diaphragm spasm. The diaphragm is the large muscle which separates the chest from the abdomen.	Try to breathe more rhythmically and lower down; move arms up and down rather than across your body.

11

**The Swim
For
Lunch Bunch**

THE SWIM FOR LUNCH BUNCH

Swimming is one of the most popular and heathful sports. Every year millions of people enjoy swimming in oceans, lakes, and rivers in all parts of the world. Plus, indoor pools in schools and recreation centers make swimming a year-round sport.

Organized swimming contests began in Great Britain during the 1880's. In the United States athletic clubs first held swimming meets in the early 1900's. Today thousands of swimmers compete in meets held by high schools, colleges, and swimming clubs throughout the United States. There are also numerous people involved in swimming for overall fitness and health. One such group in Tallahassee, Florida, is called the "Swim for Lunch Bunch."

The group was organized in 1968 by Elizabeth Barrow. Since then the group has grown to over fifty people, the majority of whom are over twenty-five years old. On most nice days you will find an average of twenty-seven people swimming during the noon hour at the Florida State University Olympic Pool.

This "Lunch Bunch" is basically a part of the AAU's Masters Swimming Program. What is Masters Swimming all about? Judge Robert E. Beach, the National Masters Swimming Vice-Chairman says, "The Masters Program is fun and health oriented. We do not want to become overly competitive. If we forget Masters Swimming is a program designed to encourage people to swim on a regular basis and to be concerned about their physical fitness, the entire program will go down the drain. It has been proven through research that no comparable physical activity can contribute to a person's well-being as much as swimming. In swimming you use more muscles of your body than any other sport. The physical fitness benefits are the major selling points but the fun aspect is also important."

Swimming provides other advantages such as:
1. A type of mental and physical therapy.
2. Something the whole family can participate in.
3. Confidence and character.
4. A lifetime sport.
5. Retardation of the aging process.
6. Insurance against heart disease.
7. Numerous health benefits.
8. Comradeship with others.

If you are interested in participating in a fitness swim club in your city, there are several rules to keep in mind, especially if you are over thirty. Captain Ransom J. Arthur, the coach of the U.S.

The Swim for Lunch Bunch

Navy Swim Team, lists these guidelines:

1. Before beginning a swim program, participants should have a complete physical exam including a blood pressure reading and electrocardiogram. They should also have a complete blood count and urinalysis. There should be no evidence in any of these studies of serious illness or defects.

2. The scheduling of the workouts should make it possible for the swimmers to take part at least three times a week. Either lunch hour or immediately after work is the best time. The workout should be no more than an hour in length.

3. Before each workout the swimmer should take a very long and hot shower to get his muscles warm and filled with blood. Similarly, the warmup prior to any kind of effort should be ample: for example, a slow swim followed by some kicks and pulls. The warmup procedure can often eliminate orthopedic difficulties such as joint and muscle problems.

4. After the long shower and warmup, the swimmer is capable of doing several timed repeats. For example, four times fifty yards with ten second's rest in between each effort is a good and safe builder of endurance. This is well-tolerated, provided the swimmer does not go in an all-out fashion but emphasizes a smooth and steady pace.

5. The workout should end in a steady swim down. After finishing the workout, another long shower is necessary with precautions taken against chilling and ear infections.

The workouts of the "Lunch Bunch" vary according to the level of the swimmer. Some of the participants swim only five hundred yards and others up to two thousand yards. The following are suggested workouts for beginning, intermediate, and advanced swimmers.

BEGINNING WORKOUT--600 yards
1 X 50 yards freestyle warmup
1 X 25 yards of kick, pull, swim, kick using freestyle
2 X 25 yards of swim, kick, pull, kick using freestyle
1 X 25 yards of each stroke: butterfly, back, breast, crawl
1 X 25 yards of each stroke: butterfly, back, breast, crawl
1 X 50 yards of freestyle work down

Kicking is when a swimmer hangs on to a kickboard and uses his legs only. Pulling is when the swimmer has his legs tied and pulls himself through the water with his arms.

The Swim for Lunch Bunch

INTERMEDIATE WORKOUT--- 1000 yards
1 X 200 yards of freestyle warmup
2 X 100 yards of medley relay swim(butterfly, back, breast, crawl)
1 X 100 yards of kick, pull, swim using individual relay
4 X 25 yards of butterfly
2 X 100 yards of freestyle work down

ADVANCED WORKOUT--- 2000 yards
1 X 200 yards of freestyle warmup
4 X 50 yards of kick, pull, swim using butterfly
8 X 25 yards using butterfy sprint
1 X 100 yards of freestyle (easy)
2 X 100 yards of kick, pull, swim using freestyle
4 X 25 yards using freestyle sprint
1 X 200 yards of freestyle workdown

Naturally, you will want to vary these schedules according to your specific needs and wants. For example, you may want to swim continuously for eight hundred yards or even a mile. Occasionally a vigorous game of water polo can also be challenging.

If you are interested in becoming more physically fit, give swimming a try. Perhaps you will soon understand why the "Swim for Lunch Bunch" makes such a big SPLASH!

12

There's a
Bicycle
Built for
You

THERE'S A BICYCLE BUILT FOR YOU

There are over eighty million bicycles being used in the United States today. The big shift from four to two wheels that happened suddenly is the result of the national pursuit of fun, fitness, sport, transportation, and ecology.

If you want to take exercise out of the "necessary evil" category and turn it into fun, then cycling is the way to do it. It provides a long list of benefits. Also, you do not have to worry about the foot and knee problems that come with jogging. (In running, each foot hits the ground with a force of from two to seven times your body weight. The faster you run, the higher the force, and force is one of the primary causes of injury. The forces are considerably less in bicycling.)

When bicycling is turned into a sport, it is as demanding and thrilling as you want it to be. As a means of transportation, it rates as a super convenience with its simplicity, size, speed, and cost. Ecologically, it remains the ultimate answer to air pollution.

The bicycle, in fact, seems destined to become a vital tool in our modern society. It does not depend on the Middle East politcal situation. It offers us a good way of getting around the whims of governments, for all we need is a couple of good legs and a conditioned body. With muscle and fitness, who needs gasoline?

For either sex, particularly for women, cycling offers one of the best body-toning activities. It involves big groups of muscles in the legs and buttocks that make up a large portion of the total body musculature.

As a method of fighting obesity, cycling has the advantage of being fun even when performed on a systematic schedule. On a vigorous ride, a cyclist can burn from 500 to 800 calories an hour.

The biggest and most important contribution of cycling, however, is heart-lung fitness. The late Dr. Paul Dudley White, famous American heart specialist, and also avid cyclist, promoted regular cycling as a good way to combat heart disease. Cycling, as a circulatory exercise, activates the internal organs—the heart, the lungs, the diaphram—in pumping more life-giving blood to the system.

Whether a bicycle becomes your perferred mode of transportation, a regular fitness activity, or a recreational pastime, you should know the following:

WHERE TO BUY A BIKE. Bike prices may vary ten dollars or more between the specialized bicycle shops and the large retail stores that deal in volumn sales but sometimes run short on quality of service. The big outlets often have inexperienced salespeople, whereas the bicycle shop has personnel trained to help you select the bike that is right for you. These shops also feature qualified mechanics who will assemble and service your bike. Proper wheel alignment, screw adjustments on chainwheels, setting the cables, and calibrating the brakes should be left to experts. It is safer.

WHAT KIND OF BIKE TO BUY. The kind of bike you buy depends on where you decide to ride. If you are merely going to be riding in your neighborhood, without any hills to consider, then a simple, balloon-tire, coaster-brake bike will be adequate. A decent one can be bought for $50. Check it over carefully before taking it on the road: frame, wheels and spokes, brakes, fenders, tires, chains.

You will need a change of gears if your terrain has gentle inclines. For going to school or the grocery store, or for taking a simple workout on a bike, an uncomplicated three-speed gives you everything you need. Good ones range in price from $60 to $90. All in all, you will probably find that the three-speed bicycle is your best buy.

If you are the adventurous type, then you will want a higher speed bike. Five-speeds give you all the power you need to climb hills on country roads. Plus, they shift smoother, are lighter in weight, and easier to handle than a three-speed. Their price starts at about $85.

The urge to buy a ten-speed can be strong when you first lay your eyes on the exotic assortment of chains and gears. For the average woman, who is simply interested in fitness, a less complex bike will prove much more enjoyable. However, for the ultimate cyclist, who covers long distances over hilly terrains, this multigeared bike is a necessity. With its doubleshift levers and front and rear *derailleurs*, it offers what you need on the straightaways, down-shifting for going up steep hills, and elimination of constant braking when going downhill. Most good ten-speeds start at $100 and can go as high as $700 for the custom-made European models.

The money you put into a bike depends on how serious you are about cycling. If you plan on becoming an advanced rider, get the best you can afford. High levels of fitness for most women, however, can be obtained on bicycles with balloon tires and coaster brakes, or simple three-speeds.

FRAMES, BRAKES, AND TIRES. A man's bike frame with its horizontal top bar is inherently stronger than a woman's. Since you will probably be riding in pants or shorts, the top bar will be no inconvenience; therefore, you should consider getting a man's bike frame.

If you have a single-speed bike, you get coaster brakes, the kind you have to back pedal to use. The multi-speed bikes all have caliper brakes, hand operated from the handbars, with the brake shoe that works by friction on the rims of the wheels. Mainly, look for both front and rear braking systems.

For all-around riding comfort, the heavier weight tires with tubes are recommended. A bit harder to change than light-weight tubeless "sew-ups," they not only withstand the beating from gravel and rough riding; but also, they are cheaper.

BIKE SIZE. Selecting the right size of bike is important. If it is too small, you will not get the full drive from your legs. If it is too large, it can be dangerous. For most women, the twenty-four to twenty-six inch bike(wheel size) will usually prove suitable. Be sure to try it for size before you buy.

Sit on the bike in your stocking feet. Place your heel on the pedal in the down position. If the bike fits, your leg should be straight. Adjust the seat height as necessary, but not more than three inches above the bolt connecting it to the frame. A seat too high causes an inbalance and creates stresses on the frame. It also makes steering and pedaling difficult.

HOW TO ADJUST YOUR BIKE. First, your bike should permit both your feet to fully and comfortably meet the ground when you straddle the crossbar. Then, while sitting squarely in the saddle(seat) with the pedal rotated to the vertical six o'clock position, make any adjustments in saddle height that permit the heel to touch the pedal with the leg fully extended. You should be able to do this with either leg without shifting your weight in the saddle.

Now, the handlebars can be adjusted so that the hand grips are at the same level as the saddle. If less than three inches of handlebar stem and seat post remain telescoped into the frame, you may have the wrong sized bike. Too high an adjustment may cause the frame to wobble, shift your balance incorrectly, and make riding dangerous.

The saddle may be adjusted forward or backward to the most comfortable postion. The body inclines forward with the arms extended to the handlebar grips. In this position, much of your body is brought into play in a coordinated rhythmic motion.

For maximum riding proficiency, the position of the foot on the pedal is a paramount importance. Avoid pedaling flat-footed with the pedal at the instep. This results in a big loss of efficiency. The secret of pedaling lies in complete spin-around action. That is, the action is not just simply a case of pushing down. Rather, by extending the foot at the ankle at the bottom of the stroke, additional power is exerted.

Then, in continuing the stroke, bring the foot back up in a circular rhythmetic motion. The ankle continually works in a coordinated extending and flexing manner. Toe stirrups attached to the pedals greatly aid this process.

If you have never been on a bike, lower the seat so that both feet touch the ground as you sit in the saddle. Now, by "scootering" yourself along with your feet, you can learn to steer and keep your balance without spilling. It will not take long. You will find when the bike is in motion, it literally steers itself and balance is easy. The worst way to learn is to have someone pushing you from behind.

CYCLING PROGRAMS. Like any other activity, cycling becomes more interesting if it has a purpose or goal. Following are eighteen-week training programs that can be used with a coaster bike or multi-speed bike. Both programs start at a beginning level and progress to the intermediate level.

CYCLING PROGRAM (BALLOON TIRE—COASTER BRAKE)

Week	Week
1. 1¼-1½ miles in 7 minutes	10. 3¾-4 miles in 20 minutes
2. 1½-1¾ miles in 8 minutes	11. 4-4¼ miles in 20 minutes
3. 1¾-2 miles in 10 minutes	12. 4¼-4½ miles in 22 minutes
4. 2-2¼ miles in 11 minutes	13. 4½-4¾ miles in 22 minutes
5. 2¼-2½ miles in 12 minutes	14. 4¾-5 miles in 25 minutes
6. 2½-2¾ miles in 13 minutes	15. 5-5¼ miles in 25 minutes
7. 2¾-3 miles in 14 minutes	16. 5¼-5½ miles in 27 minutes
8. 3-3½ miles in 16 minutes	17. 5½-6 miles in 30 minutes
9. 3½-3¾ miles in 18 minutes	18. 6½ miles in 30 minutes

Start on level one and spend one week at each level, or eighteen weeks in all. You should ride three or four days a week. When level eighteen is reached, three days a week is sufficient. By this time, you should be well on your way to obtaining a high level of fitness.

CYCLING PROGRAM (MULTI-SPEED)

Week	Week
1. 2 miles in 7½ minutes	10. 5 miles in 18½ minutes
2. 2 miles in 7 minutes	11. 6 miles in 23 minutes
3. 3 miles in 12 minutes	12. 6 miles in 22½ minutes
4. 3 miles in 11½ minutes	13. 6 miles in 22 minutes
5. 4 miles in 15½ minutes	14. 7 miles in 27 minutes
6. 4 miles in 15 minutes	15. 7 miles in 26½ minutes
7. 4 miles in 14½ minutes	16. 7 miles in 26 minutes
8. 5 miles in 19½ minutes	17. 8 miles in 31 minutes
9. 5 miles in 19 minutes	18. 8 miles in 29-30 minutes

Of course, occasionally, you can vary from this set cycling pattern. For example, on a weekend you may want to take a five or ten mile joyride. Or, you may want to lead the whole family in a bicycling outing.

Once you have gotten the nine or ten weeks of programmed effort behind you, you will see the real meaning of cycling. You will ride comfortably without fatigue or soreness. You will look forward to your next workout. You will see excess body fat disappear and your muscles taking on pleasing contours. In short, you will be ready for a lifetime of fun and fitness. HAPPY CYCLING!

Misconceptions
about Exercise

13

MISCONCEPTIONS ABOUT EXERCISE

Almost everyone has theories about exercise: how to—how not to—when to—how much—why.

Where do these theories come from? Many come from our parents, friends, teachers, and coaches. Some are simply general hand-me-down folklore and cleverly designed advertisements. This is fine if most of them are based on sound, physiological facts. In reality, though, at least three out of four of these theories are based on ignorance and false beliefs. Here are just a few of these misconceptions.

Running is the best all-around exercise for fitness.

Before you can decide what is the best all-around exercise for fitness, it's necessary to answer the question: fitness for what? The same degree of physical fitness is not necessary for everyone. Your fitness should be sufficient to meet the requirements for your job, plus a little extra reserve for emergencies. A basketball player or diver needs a different type of physical fitness than that required by a housewife or a secretary. While running is a good exercise, so are swimming, bicycling, and tennis. It should be clearly understood, though, that running is bad for some people, especially those who have joint problems.

Therefore, to decide what the "the best" exercise is, you must determine your own needs and wants. Age and medical problems are also considerations.

Exercise causes weight loss.

If you expect to lose weight by simply exercising, you will probably be disappointed. Not that exercise isn't important in losing weight. It is, but that's just part of the story. Diet is the other part.

For example, if over a period you eat the caloric amount of food you need to replace the energy you use, your weight will remain about the same. If you eat more food than you need, you will gain weight unless your physical activity increases proportionately. On the other hand, if you cut down on calories as you continue to exercise, you will lose weight.

Remember, both DIET and EXERCISE are important in weight control.

Strenuous exercise is bad for the heart

This is a double misconception based on the notions that the enlarged heart of the athlete is a condition to be avoided and that strenuous exercise can damage a healthy heart. There is such a condition as an unhealthy enlarged heart, but it bears no resemblance to the athlete's heart. Like any other muscle that is exercised, the heart tends to become larger, stronger, and more efficient. The fear that strenuous exercise causes heart damage is unfounded. Medical authorities tell us that the other muscles will tire-out during physical activity long before a healthy heart can be adversely affected.

Vigorous stretching exercises keep your muscles flexible.
Vigorous stretching actually causes your muscles to contract, rather than relax. Therefore all stretching exercises should be done slowly, smoothly, and carefully, with special emphasis on avoiding jerky or bouncy movements.

For example, if you want to stretch the hamstrings—-the muscles in the back of your thighs—-you should sit on the floor, legs in front of you, and bend forward to try to touch your toes. Move slowly. When the first sigh of pain occurs, hold that position for several seconds, then relax. Repeat this movement several times.

What usually happens, however, is that most people, in an attempt to touch their toes, will start bobbing and bouncing. Not only is this counter-productive, it is actually dangerous.

There is a sensor system (called the stretch reflex) in each muscle that automatically reacts to a sudden stretch. This is a way of protecting against overstretching. Whenever you bounce forward, quickly pulling the hamstrings, a reflex contraction occurs that inhibits elongation. By bouncing, you actually keep the muscles from relaxing enough to extend to their full capacity. And, if force is applied, parts of the muscle can be overstretched and torn.

So—- in practicing stretching movements, make sure you do them SLOWLY and SMOOTHLY.

Women should avoid exercise because it will develop big muscles.
This is another common misconception. The average woman could not develop large muscles if her life depended upon it. Why? Because she does not have enough of the masculine hormones that are necessary for this process to take place. The fact that some women do have muscular legs only means that they inherited this trait, not that they developed these muscles as a result of a particular exercise

or activity.

Generally speaking, women should practice the same basic exercise program that men do.

Proper exercise is time consuming.

Most people can improve their physical fitness with as little as five or ten minutes at a time. This means a time allotment of one or two hours a week for exercise. You can look at it this way: allowing eight hours a night for sleeping, you still have 112 hours a week left over. Who can honestly say that devoting one or two of them to exercise would seriously curtail any other activities?

Weight training is good for the skeletal muscles, but not the heart.

While numerous people recognize the value of weight training in developing strength in the skeletal muscles, they assume it has little or no value in exercising the heart. This is simply not true. Weight training can definitely have a stimulating effect on the heart, especially if large muscle exercises are performed for ten to twelve repetitions with little rest between exercises.

The older you are, the less you need exercise.

Older women need exercise as much, perhaps even more, than younger ones, who are less apt to be troubled with stiffening joints and poor circulation. The kind of activity a woman undertakes, however, should be suitable to her strength and state of health. Generally, it is a good idea to lessen the intensity of exercise with each passing decade, but at the same time the quanity can be increased. As a rule, the older a woman grows, the more sedentary she tends to become, and the more she need exercise.

Exercise increases your need for protein foods.

Many people assume that vigorous physical activity results in protein loss because of "wear and tear" on the muscles. But if this assumption were true, the body, in breaking down the protein molecules, would excrete nitrogen in the form of urea. Numerous experiments in nitrogen balance indicate that the amount of nitrogen the body excretes after vigorous exercise is not significantly higher than the amounts excreted after the body has been resting.

People who exercise should stick to a well-balanced diet composed of a wide variety of foods and not concentrate on just protein-rich foods.

Misconceptions About Exercise

You should work up a good sweat during an exercise period.

While exercising we produce heat in proportion to the amount of muscle activity. The body's temperature could easily rise as much as ten degrees F or more, if this heat were not dissipated. Fortunately, the body is designed to keep itself from overheating. Warm blood is brought to the skin where it loses heat to the surrounding air. The sweat glands begin to secrete water, and the body is further cooled by evaporation of the perspiration. In cold weather, heat is given off easily. But in hot weather the body must sweat profusely in order to cool itself.

So, it should be obvious that sweating does not do anything but lower the body temperature. It does not help reduce body fat. You may weigh less after a workout, but this is due to loss of water, and there is very little water in fat. As soon as you quench your thirst, you will gain the lost weight back.

Sweating does not "clean out your pores" either. There is no evidence that it is of any value in removing toxic materials from the body. For this reason, you should avoid rubber sweat suits, belts, and wraps. Even steam and sauna baths can lead to problems rather than fitness.

Sweating does not promote fitness. Fitness is developed by exercising the muscles of the body—not the sweat glands.

Children do not need regular exercise.

The average child does need regular exercise. Even though he starts out more than active enough to maintain a state of physical fitness, his activity tends to dwindle as time goes by. The average overweight child who often shies away from participation in active games is even more in need of regular exercise. Also, children need to develop skills in individual and dual sports that will carry over into their adulthoods.

Therefore, regular and supervised programs of exercise and physical education are important components of a child's life.

Exercise will benefit your body but not your brain.

While research definitely proves that exercise benefits the body, recent findings suggest that exercise plays an important part in improving mental performance. Studies have shown that exercise can increase the oxygen-transport capacity to all parts of the body, including the brain. Early research demonstrated that brain cells deprived of sufficient oxygen do not perform their work efficiently, and the intellect and reasoning powers fail as a result. Thus, these studies demonstrate that a program of regular exercise that increases oxygen transport to the brain can significantly improve mental performance. For optimum results, however, exercise should be varied and challenging, and not just routine and repetitous.

It is dangerous for pregnant women to exercise.

Exercise kept within sensible bounds presents no threat to a pregnant woman as long as she is free from conditions that would, in the estimation of her obstetrician, rule exercise out. Sensible exercise, in fact, offers the pregnant woman the added advantage of toning and strengthening her lower back, buttock, and abdominal muscles, which must perform during birth. Many times the backaches that frequently follow childbirth can be prevented with proper exercise.

Exercising once in a while is better than not exercising at all.

If you do not exercise regularly, say exercise physiologists, you are better off not attempting an exercise program at all. Occasional strenuous activity can subject your body to undue strain and stress, as your body is only accustomed to inactivity. Unless you can exercise at least twice a week, stay away from the Sunday afternoon game of softball or tennis. Exercise should be an integral part of every man's and woman's life. You will feel better and look better if you make it part of your lifestyle.

Massage is the best way to get rid of cellulite.

Chances are you have been bombarded lately with magazine and TV ads alerting you to the dangers of cellulite. This is just what I was speaking of as "cleverly designed advertisements." Supposedly, it is a special type of hard-to-remove fat that can only be eliminated by costly and elaborate programs---many of which include massage.

First of all, there are no special types of fat. Fat is fat whether it is dimpled, bumpy, or looks like orange peel. To put it concisely, there is no such thing as cellulite. The American Medical Association issued a statement calling cellulite a hoax and denouncing its remedies as economic exploitation. To make matters worse, there have been reports of women seriously injured by types of treatments used such as deep bruising massage, sweat inducing body wraps, hormone injections, and starvation diets.

As for massage, it may be relaxing and make you feel good, but it will not remove fat. It is impossible to push it off or shake it off. Sorry!

Other than fatty tumors (lipomas) the right treatment for unwanted fat is directed toward eliminating obesity. Since spot reducing is not possible, you must gradually lose fat from all over your body. That means good diet habits (no fads or crash efforts, but a sensible, regular, well-balanced diet) and proper exercise.

14

How to Keep in Shape
During Pregnancy

HOW TO KEEP IN SHAPE DURING PREGNANCY

What do exercise and muscle have to do with pregnancy and birth? Probably a lot more than you realize. Read on for complete details.

Congratulations! So you are planning on having a baby.

The happy expectant prenatal period of a woman's life need not be a period of passiveness. In fact, just the oppposite should be true.

The mother-to-be, whether it is for the first or the fifth time, should be in the best of health in order to enjoy her normal recreational endeavors and continue her daily activities. This is the time when a woman should pay the most attention to exercise.

There are many good reasons why exercise is important during pregnancy. All of them center around the basic relationship between exercise and muscle. Simply stated, the relationship is as follows: exercise, properly performed, increases the strength and endurance of muscles, the flexibility of muscles, and the tone of muscles as well as the body's heart-circulatory efficiency.

The points below should help clarify some of the specific relationships of exercise, muscles, and pregnancy.

Birth involves the relaxation and contraction of many major muscle groups (the uterus, abdominal, buttock, thigh). If these muscles are in good condition, you will have an easier time at birth. Also, you will feel and look better---before and after the baby is born.

Prior to birth, especially during the last trimester, there is extra stress and strain on certain muscles. For example toward the end of pregnancy, many women tilt their pelvic area forward and bend the upper part of their bodies backward to compensate for the weight of the heavy uterus. As a result, backache frequently develops. As breasts become larger, additonal stress is placed on the underlying support muscles: the chest (pectoralis major), the shoulder (deltoid), and even the upper back (trapezius).

The increasing needs of pregnancy put an added burden on a mother's heart. Proper exercise can increase your heart's efficiency.

There is also a slowing of the blood flow in the lower extremities during pregnancy. Many times this can cause stagnation of the blood in the legs which leads to varicose veins. Exercise will improve your circulation.

Pregancy also disturbs the gastrointestinal tract. This can result in constipation and hemorroids. Proper exercise can assist by providing tone and massage to the intestinal tract.

127

Exercise causes your body to burn calories at a higher than normal rate. Thus, you can consume more nutritious food and still not add excess body fat.

If you establish sensible exercise habits during pregnancy, they will

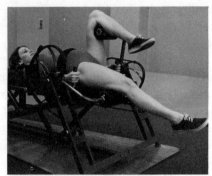

Hip and Back Machine

carry over into your everyday life style. Hopefully, these habits will provide positive examples for your children to follow.

To further convince you of the importance of good muscles to a happy,healthy pregnancy, here are a few additional facts.

Your body contains three types of muscles: the voluntary or skeletal muscles, the involuntary muscles such as those of the digestive tract, and the heart muscle. Our movement potential is brought into action by 434 skeletal muscles. They are composed of 250 million smaller units, the muscles fibers, and make up 32% of the weight of typical American female. It is important to know muscles are arranged in pairs. One set of muscles is on one side of the joint for bending at the joint. On the other side of the joint is another set for straightening the joint. A good example are the muscles of the upper arm. These muscles bend and straighten the arm at the joint of the elbow.The muscles in front of the elbow joint, primarily the biceps, bend the arm. The muscles in the rear of the elbow, the triceps, straighten the arm. Similar situations exist on both sides of all joints, although many are more complex than the muscles involved in the movement around the elbow joint. Depending on the desired direction of movement at the moment, these opposite-working sets of muscles are called

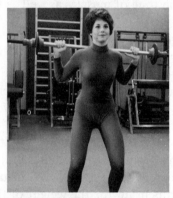

Wide squat

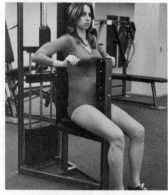

Rowing Machine

either agonist muscles or antagonist muscles. An agonist muscle produces movement by contraction. An antagonist muscle limits or stops movement by refusing to permit itself to be stretched.

In order for movement to occur, an agonist muscle must reduce its length, contract with a pulling force that produces movement; but simultaneously, the antagonist muscle must permit movement by allowing its length to be increased. Thus, during all movements, while one set of muscles is getting shorter, another set of muscles must be getting longer.

The point of the last paragraphs is to show that a muscle produces movement by synchonized contraction and relaxation.

In much the same way, the birth process, although partially controlled by hormones and involuntary muscles, is still greatly assisted by the strength and flexibility of the skeletal muscles. In fact, during labor and delivery, most muscles in your body work to capacity. It is vital that you improve your ability to contract and relax your muscles. How can you do this? Exercise, of course!

EXERCISE: WHAT KIND? HOW MUCH?

While pregnancy and birth involve most muscle groups to some degree, the primary muscles affected are the abdominals, buttocks, lower back, and chest. Special attention should be given to these areas. But, at the same time, your other muscle groups (thighs, calves, shoulders, upper back, and arms) should not be neglected.

The recommended exercises are divided into two groups. The first group is done with equipment that is frequently found in athletic clubs or training centers. The second group is composed of barbell and free-hand exercises.

Nautilus Machine Exercises	Barbell/Free-hand Exercises
1. Hip and Back	1. Wide squat
2. Leg Extension	2. Pelvic raise
3. Calf raise on Multi-Exercise	3. Calf raise
4. Pullover	4. Pullover
5. Rowing	5. Shoulder shrug
6. Double chest	6. Bench press
7. Negative-accentuated sit-up	7. Negative-accentuated sit-up

Properly performed, you can get good results from the barbell and free-hand exercises. But you get much better results from using the Nautilus machines. The Nautilus machines are scientifically designed to provide full-range exercises.

129

NAUTILUS MACHINE EXERCISES

Photos on the Nautilus Machine are of Mrs. Patricia Sauers. Mrs. Sauers was eight months pregnant when she demonstrated these exercises. She is now the mother of a robust boy.

1. HIP AND BACK MACHINE. Direct resistance for the large muscles of your buttocks and lower back is provided in this movement. A repetition is completed when the legs are straight with the lower back arched and the buttocks tightened. The photo illustrates the alternating leg style that is used.

2. LEG EXTENSION MACHINE. From this position, the legs are smoothly extended. After a brief pause, the resistance should be slowly lowered and repeated. You will feel this exercise in your frontal thigh muscles.

3. PULLOVER MACHINE. This is a great exercise for your torso muscles. The photo shows the stretched, starting position. From here your elbows are rotated down until the pads are behind your waist. Pause, slowly return to the starting position and repeat.

4. ROWING MACHINE. Many women have problems with their posture during pregnancy. This exercise will solve that common problem by strengthening the upper back and shoulder muscles. The picture shows Mrs. Sauer in the contracted position of this exercise.

5. DOUBLE CHEST MACHINE. Two exercises are performed on this machine. Arm Crosses immediately followed by Decline Presses. The photo shows the contracted position of the primary movement of the Arm Crosses. The next photo shows the contracted position of the secondary movement, the Decline Press.

BARBELL/FREE-HAND EXERCISES

The barbell/freehand exercises are demonstrated by Mrs. Deborah Myhand. These photographs were taken shortly after Mrs. Myhand gave birth to a healthy girl.

How to Keep in Shape During Pregnancy

1. WIDE SQUAT. With hands on your hips, or barbell on your shoulders, and feet about eighteen inches apart (see photo), slowly descend to full-squat position. Keep your head up and torso erect as you stand up and repeat. Do not bounce at the bottom. Keep the movements steady and controlled. The squat will strengthen your thighs and buttocks.

2. PELVIC RAISE. Assume a supine position as shown in the photograph. Raise hips as high as possible. Pause, arch your back, and tighten your buttocks—then slowly lower to the starting position and repeat.

3. CALF RAISE. For this exercise you will need a pad or board to stand on and a small bench to rest your arms on. From the position shown in the photograph, slowly lower and raise your heels as much as possible. Be sure to stretch as far down as you can and keep your knees locked throughout the movement.

4. PULLOVER. A small bench and a 2 1/2 or 5 pound weight will be needed for this exercise. Get into the position that is pictured. Keep your arms straight as you pull the weight over your head until your arms are perpendicular to the floor. Slowly lower your arms, stretch, and repeat.

5. SHOULDER SHRUG. Securely grasp a light barbell and stand. Keeping your arms straight, shrug your shoulders as high as possible trying to touch your ears. Pause, slowly lower, and repeat. This exercise will strengthen your upper back and shoulders.

6. BENCH PRESS. You will need someone to help you with this movement. Have your helper hand you a light barbell when you are securely situated on the bench. Slowly bend your arms until the barbell touches your chest, and press the barbell in a controlled manner to the straight-arm position. Pause and repeat.

7. NEGATIVE-ACCENTUATED SIT-UP. With your knees bent, toes securely held down, hands on your waist (see photo), slowly lower your torso until your back touches the floor. Use your hands to assist you in the sitting-up process and repeat. You will feel this in your stomach muscles.

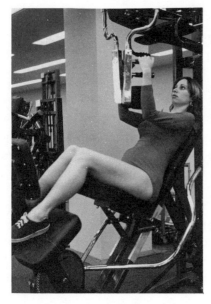

Double Chest Machine (1)

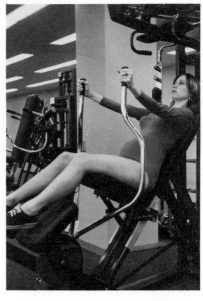

Double Chest Machine (2)

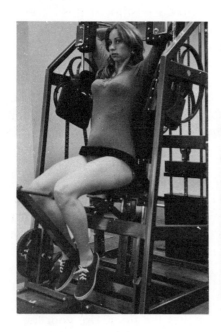

Pullover Machine

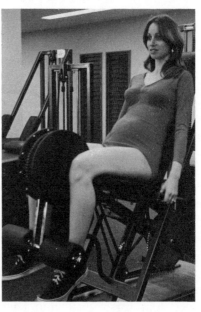

Leg Extension Machine

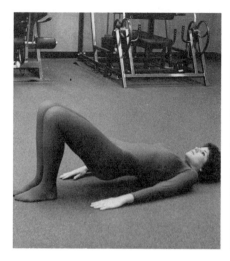

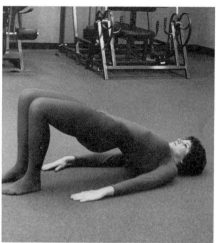

Pelvic raise (starting)   **Pelvic raise (contracted)**

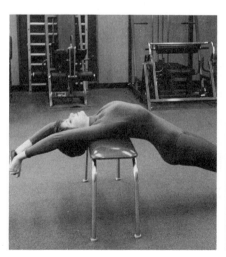

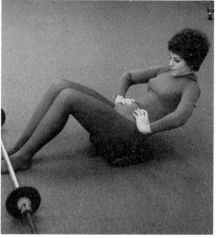

Pullover   **Negative-accentuated sit-up**

133

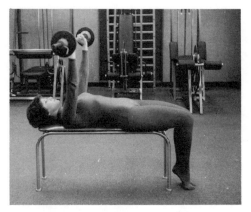

Bench press (1)

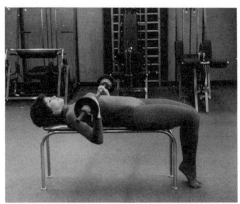

Bench press (2)

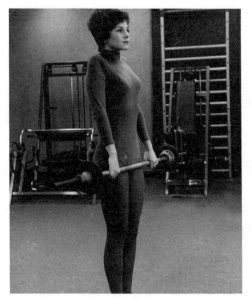

Shoulder shrug

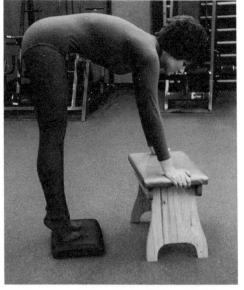

Calf raise

How to Keep in Shape During Pregnancy

There are some frequently asked questions which I would like to take this opportunity to answer.

Will regular exercise make childbirth easier? To answer this question with a "yes" requires no more than common sense according to Dr. Clayton Thomas. "If you could separate all the people on the earth into those who exercise and those who do not, who do you think would be the healthiest and have the easiest time having babies? It would be a paradox if a sedentary person had fewer problems. I know of no evidence that exercise is harmful in pregnancy."

I compete in women's athletics. Now I am pregnant, how will this affect my abilities? Should I discontinue my competition altogether? Noticeable changes in athletic performance first show up at the end of the third month. Most mothers gain only about three pounds the first trimester, but in the second trimester, the uterus expands twenty times, and a woman will gain about ten pounds. The extra weight, protruding stomach, a loss of balance, the effects of water retention and anemia, may simply make competition effort too complicated. Even the well-trained athlete may find it difficult to do her best at this point.

Because of the deterioration of performance, most athletes give up competition, but not exercise, by the third month, although a woman who is used to competition and heavy training could safely compete beyond this time. Physicians get a bit alarmed when they hear of these efforts and recommend that athletes not compete too far into pregnancy, stopping by the sixth month. But, there is no hard evidence that competition during pregnancy is harmful, and a woman should judge by the way she feels when it is time to quit.

Will having a baby ruin my athletic ability? Considering the number of women who have broken world records and won prizes in major competitions, it is hard to understand how people still believe the myth that having a baby will ruin an athlete. For example, Madeliene Manning won a gold medal in the 800 meters in the 1968 Olympics, then got married and had a baby. In 1972 she broke her own record in the Games that year. Then, there is professional tennis star Margaret Court. In 1971, when Court announced that she was leaving the tennis circuit until after the birth of her first child, most followers thought she was through for good. The next year following the birth of her baby, she won twenty-three out of twenty-six tournaments and over $200,000 to become one of the highest female money winners of all time.

Exactly what is a miscarriage? Is there danger of a miscarriage if I compete in compete in vigorous sports? A miscarriage means that the fetus is born before it is capable of surviving outside of a mother's body. The majority of miscarriages occur during the second or third month of pregnancy while a small number carry through to the seventh month. In microscopic examinations of miscarried embryos and fetuses, more than 80% reveal a deformity or biological malfunction that would make it impossible for the baby to survive and live a normal life. A miscarriage, in most instances, should be considered one of nature's own built-in check valves.

There is very little danger of miscarriage from vigorous sport activity, especially if you are accustomed to that activity. Why? Because the fetus is well-cushioned. It floats in a sac of fluid that works like a shock absorber. Therefore, you cannot jiggle a baby loose by running, jumping, or horseback riding. Nor can you harm it by swimming. Very strong stomach blows or falls in the eighth or ninth month might start labor contractions prematurely, so physicians advise against vigorous sports or contact sports toward the end of pregnancy.

What kind of program should I follow after my baby is born? Unless your physician advises you otherwise, or barring unusual complications, you may begin simple exercise while you are in the hospital. Try to do it daily, once or twice at first, with gradual increases in repetitions. I would suggest these exercises for the first week:

Leg raise and tuck. Lie flat on your back. Keeping your left leg straight, raise your right foot off the bed about six inches. Now bend your right knee smoothly, then straighten, and lower. Do the same with the left leg.

After the first week of performing this simple exercise, and once you are home, you can begin free-hand exercises that you became accustomed to during your pregnancy.

I recommend the squat, pelvic raise, calf raise, and negative-accentuated sit-up. You should do them daily with gradual increases in repetitions for the next two weeks.

By the end of the third week, you may begin some light walking and add the barbell or Nautilus machine exercises to your routine.

After another week—four weeks after the baby was born—you should be ready to get back into your previous routine: resistance exercises every other day, with brisk walking in between.

The average woman spends six weeks resting up before getting back into a routine. Most well-conditioned women are able to start training in four weeks, and usually no more than six.

Does every woman get stretch marks? What can I do about them? Stretch marks, which often appear on the breasts and abdomen during pregnancy, are due to the tearing of elastic tissues in the skin that accompanies enlargement of the breasts, distention of the abdomen, and deposition of subcultaneous fat. They are pink or purplish-red lines during pregnancy. The lines become a permanent grayish-white scarlike marks after delivery. Some women never develop stretch marks despite bearing several children; others lose most of the tone of their skin after one pregnancy (evidently there is an inherited factor involved). Stretch marks cannot be considered evidence that a woman has borne a child, however, because they are seen on women who have not been pregnant.

Once you get stretch marks, there is nothing you can do about them. You might help to prevent them by being sure that you do not gain excessive amounts of body fat and that you adhere to a well-balanced diet.

How are varicose veins related to pregnancy? Varicose veins are bulging, twisted, and knotted veins that are usually located right under the skin. While they frequently occur in pregnant women, they also appear in other women and men as well. Most often they develop in the legs, although they can pop out other places like the anal area (hemorroids) and the genital area. Their presence is due to two factors. One, many pregnancies contribute to a generally weakened condition of the veins in the legs if the pressure created by the baby cuts off some of the circulation. Two, varicose veins can be inherited. In such a case, the individual probably inherited a tendency toward inelasticity in the wall veins.

In both instances, however, the results are the same: there is a weakness or malfunction within the flaplike valves of the vein. As the weight of the blood on the vein wall increases, the vein bulges, and after long stretching, it loses its elasticity and finally becomes elongated, twisted, and knotted.

Will exercise help varicose veins? Yes. Any type of contracting or pumping of the leg muscles helps to literally milk the blood out of the calves and thighs and propel it upward toward the heart. Brisk walking is a good exercise, and calf raises and squats are even better. Everyone can benefit by maintaining good muscle tone in the thigh and calf muscles. The strong, firm muscles around deep veins help provide external support and help protect them from overstretching and damage.

Can varicose veins be prevented? If you have inherited a tendency toward varicose veins, you probably will not be able to prevent them. The following measures though will help to minimize them:

1. Don't stand for long periods. If you must, wear lightweight support stockings. When standing on the bus, at your job, or at the kitchen sink, flex your toes every few minutes and then rise slowly on your tiptoes.

2. Don't sit for long periods, especially with your legs crossed. When sitting, elevate your legs or change their position. On long train, plane, or bus trips walk about every half hour. On long car trips, switch drivers frequently or stop for light exercise every hour if possible.

3. Avoid tight garments that constrict your legs: girdles, garters, and knee-high stockings. High boots with elastic around the top are especially bad.

4. Keep your body weight within a normal range.

Are there other precautions I should take to prevent varicose veins from getting worse? Yes, in addition to the ones listed above:

1. Wear support stockings. They counteract the pressure of the blood against the vein walls.

2. Elevate your legs at least twice a day for thirty minutes. Use one or two pillows under your calves so that your legs are above the level of your heart. Be sure your knees are bent.

3. Be careful to avoid bumping, bruising, or scratching your legs since phlebitis may result.

4. Prevent skin infections on the feet and legs; they could cause serious complications. This is particularly true if you are a diabetic. Wash your feet daily, making sure you get between the toes. After bathing, apply lanolin or baby oil if you have dry skin. If your feet perspire, apply a non-medicated talcum powder. Be sure to get this between your toes.

5. Take long walks and exercise regularly. When you walk briskly (wearing support stockings), the muscles in your legs milk the veins, aiding the return of blood to the heart.

CONCLUSION

Exercise during your pregnancy can help you and your baby be healthier. A sensible exercise program can also help with the problem of varicose veins. Although it cannot cure varicose veins, it can certainly help them. By following the above suggestions, you will not only keep in shape during pregnancy, you will be in better shape after your pregnancy!

15

**Fatigue:
What Do You
Really
Know about It?**

FATIGUE: WHAT DO YOU REALLY KNOW ABOUT IT?

No one likes to have that tired, run-down feeling. In fact, formulas for how to avoid it and how to relieve it have always been eagerly sought. Much of the formula, in my opinion, involves a basic understanding of fatigue.

WHAT IS FATIGUE?

Although fatigue implies tiredness and inability to continue, it is difficult to define. The most common definition given is that fatigue is the decrease in work capacity as a result of work itself. In other words, it is the loss of use owing to use. The applies equally to physical, emotional, and mental fatigue.

Different types of work and exercise produce different types of muscular fatigue. For example, after a 100-yard dash, you will have difficulty moving your legs. Why? Because they're clogged with waste products—mostly lactic acid—that have accumulated as a result of use.

On the other hand, at the end of a long day of snow skiing, the loss of use of your legs may be due to having used up all available fuel. This is sometimes called the "fatigue of exhaustion." By contrast the former is called the "fatigue of depression." This is because the chemical reactions necessary to muscular function are depressed by accumulated waste products.

An illustration will help. A fire may go out for two reasons: either all the fuel may be consumed (exhaustion) or the grate may be clogged with much unburned coal left. In the latter case, the fire was choked out or depressed, probably owing to lack of draft. Actually, both conditions always exist in part, simutaneously. Likewise, fatigue is always due partly to exhaustion and partly to depression. The proportion of each varies. In a long, sustained effort, exhaustion predominates; in a short, intense effort, depression predominates.

WHAT IS MEANT BY MENTAL FATIGUE?

Mental fatigue is due to excessive mental activity. It shows itself in boredom; in skipping memory, in wavering attention, or inability to concentrate on a problem; in sleepiness; in failure to find the right word; in mispronunciations and all kinds of inaccuracies and mistakes; in loss of fine coordination movements of tongue and hand; and in change of temperament, such as carelessness, grouchiness, general irritability, and loss of temper.

140

WHAT IS THE BEST REMEDY FOR MENTAL FATIGUE?

The best remedy is sleep and recreational activity that does not demand too much thinking. Often, a moderately strenuous team sport is a good choice. It should provide an opportunity to forget and also provide circulation. This will promote sleep. Bridge or a game of chess, on the other hand, is hardly the best recreation for an overworked brain.

WHAT IS MEANT BY EMOTIONAL FATIGUE?

Emotional fatigue is due to excessive worry, anxiety, fear, or sexual excitment. During all kinds of intense emotions—be they love or hate— there are marked changes, particularly in heart, blood vessels, stomach, and intestines. These show themselves in loss of appetite, upset stomach, diarrhea, and sometimes constipation. The heart beats fast; the blood pressure rises; the skin may become clammy with sweat; and there is a frequent desire to urinate without real need.

When these emotional effects are long continued or often repeated, they upset the nutritive machinery of the body. Consequently, there is a loss of weight and often a lowered resistance to disease.

Long-continued worries of all kinds produce nervousness and, in extreme cases, may lead to a nervous breakdown. This breakdown occurs when the mind gives up trying to solve the problems that brought them on.

HOW CAN WORRIES BE OVERCOME?

It is very hard to stop thinking the thoughts that are associated with strong emotions, such as love, anger, fear, and hate. Two methods of overcoming worries are:

1. Escape by replacement.--This is done by finding some other activity that demands complete attention and makes it impossible to keep thinking of your worries. A game of tennis, golf, or the movies, or some form of dancing may prove satisfactory.

2. Dissolution of the emotions.--Sometimes this method needs the help of a trained counselor or psychiatrist. Often, though, it can be done by discussing your innermost worries with a trusted friend or thinking through the cause of these worries and then associating other ideas and emotions with them.

WHAT CAN BE DONE ABOUT FATIGUE?

All forms of fatigue can be overcome by rest. For mental and especially emotional fatigue, it is very hard to secure rest because the mind and emotions keep repeating themselves. They cannot be stopped as easily as the muscles.

IS THERE ANY ONE SPECIAL CAUSE OF FATIGUE?

No. Bodily activity is performed by a cooperation of muscles, heart, blood vessels, lungs, and nervous system. Any one of these may fail and thus bring the whole system to a halt. The rule, " a chain is as strong as its weakest link," applies here.

Often the nervous system gives out first. This may be because it is overworked or because the circulation fails to bring enough blood with oxygen to keep it going. Sometimes muscles accumulate too much acid. This, in turn, may be carried to the breathing center in the brain and make us gasp uncomfortably. Perhaps a small muscle is overtaxed. This may be the weak link that stops the whole activity.

ARE THERE WAYS TO QUICK RECOVERY FROM FATIGUE?

After exhausting muscular work, you should not flop down and completely relax. Recovery occurs more quickly if you slowly taper off the activity. That is why race horses trot around the track again after the race and trained athletes keep moving after their events. The continued exercise is necessary for good circulation to your muscles.

When fatigue is caused by the depletion of your energy supply (long-distance running or events that require continuous activity for at least forty minutes), it is important to eat carbohydrate-rich foods. Scientists have found that carbohydrate-rich foods definitely aid "fatigue of exhaustion" recovery, but only if they are consumed within the immediate ten-hour period of exhaustion. So, quick consumption is important!

IS THERE ANY WAY OF POSTPONING FATIGUE?

Strong muscles fatigue less quickly than weak muscles do, and strong hearts and lungs also last much longer. A progressive resistance program, properly performed, will strengthen your skeletal muscles, as well as improve the efficiency of your heart and lungs.

Well-balanced meals, day in and day out, will also help in postponing fatigue. Try to consume at least one serving from each of the four basic food groups (meat, dairy, fruit-vegetable, bread-cereal) at each meal.

Fatigue: What Do You Really Know about It?

WHAT REALLY MAKES MY MUSCLES ACHE?

There are several causes for aching muscles:

1. Lack of blood to a muscle can produce pain. When a muscle is fully contracted, it cuts off its own blood supply. This explains the pain when a heavy weight is held for a long time, or when a muscle or part of a muscle goes into cramps.

2. Strenuous exercise can produce soreness. This soreness usually occurs from twenty-four to forty-eight hours after exercise. No one knows exactly what produces this soreness. Perhaps it is due to a slight tear in the muscle or to a chemical change brought on by the acid waste products. Some physiologists think the soreness is not in the muscle itself but in the surrounding sheath and attachments. Nevertheless, it certainly brings several days of discomfort.

WHAT CAN DO DONE ABOUT MUSCULAR SORENESS?

Never should you completely rest the day after muscular fatigue. This actually makes the soreness worse. Whatever it is that made you sore is also the best means to relieve soreness. For example, if your legs are sore from bicycling around the lake, then additional bicyling (even though it is painful at first) will bring the best relief. However, anything that improves circulation will help. Massage---rubbing toward the heart---a hot bath, or any form of heat may prove useful.

WHY DOES JUST STANDING SOMETIMES SEEM MORE TIRING THAN VIGOROUS EXERCISE?

An important cause of fatigue is insufficient blood in the muscles and the brain. Movement is necessary to drive blood back to the heart in order that the heart, in turn, can send it to the brain and all parts of the body. In just standing, the blood gets stalled in the legs. This stagnation of blood in the legs can be overcome by slight muscular activity, such as wiggling the toes or alternately contracting and relaxing the calf muscles.

HOW CAN I HELP MYSELF FALL ASLEEP?

The following suggestion should prove helpful:

1. Light exercise near bedtime.
2. A small snack or something to drink.
3. A warm shower.
4. After retiring, practice relaxing your muscles. First tighten them, then relax.

5. Try reading, but stay away from exciting material. If it is un-interesting or hard, the mind is more likely to give up and go to sleep.

6. If you cannot sleep, by all means do not worry about it. Instead, say to yourself: "quiet rest is almost as good as sleep." Then imagine it is early morning, and you have just awakened and were wishing you did not have to get up. Then think how lucky you are you do not have to get up.

SHOULD I TAKE SALT PILLS IN HOT WEATHER TO COMBAT FATIGUE?

It is unlikely that a person who eats regular meals will ever be short of salt. Besides, salt pills can irritate your stomach or be passed completely undissolved. In excessive sweating during hot weather, more water is always lost than salt. You can combat the situation by drinking liberal amounts of liquids before, during, and after activity, and by using liberal amounts of table salts in foods.

DO "PEP PILLS" REALLY HELP?

Certain drugs related to amphetamine have the effect of improving mood, increasing wakefulness, and making one reckless. Because of their action on the brain, amphetamines have been used to treat depression, to combat fatigue, and to depress the appetite in the obese. Recently, however, they have proved to be drugs of addiction upon which you can easily become dependent, and it is known that brain damage can result from continued high doses. The use of amphetamines or "pep pills" has been discontinued in cases of fatigue, obesity, and, to a great extent, depression.

IS COFFEE GOOD FOR FATIGUE?

Coffee, tea, and cocoa all contain a group of stimulants of which caffeine is the most active. Caffeine is also found in most cola-flavored beverages. It is a useful means of remaining alert. Although the caffeine in coffee gives a temporary feeling of refreshment, it is no substitute for rest after hard work. On the negative side, caffeine acts on the kidneys, increasing the flow of urine, and on the heart, stimulating it to produce palpitations after over-indulgence. It also increases secretions and can produce gastritis and peptic ulcers.

You've Got 5 Minutes to Relax!

16

YOU'VE GOT 5 MINUTES TO RELAX!

*Here's how those 5 minute rest breaks can
become the most important 5 minutes in your life.*

The stresses and strains of today's society can be seen every-where. No one is immune from the disturbing conditions in our culture and our general way of life. Take a look at the average person on the street. Does he have a tense face, a jerky walk, poor posture, a fatigued appearance? Or, better yet, answer these questions for yourself: Do you wake up tired and listless in the morning? Do you feel irritable? Are you a chronic worrier? Do you feel rushed, as though you are always a little behind?

If you have answered "yes" to any of the above questions, read on. The next five minutes may just give you a new lease on life. With the use of several simple tricks, you can prevent some of the tension and stress that take so much of the zest out of living.

YAWNING---A ONE-MINUTE WONDER

Let's start with a one-minute trick that you can use over and over during the day---yawning. If you are the average person, your face is probably tense, your jaws clamped together, your lips are compressed, your chest feels tight, and your eyebrows are contracted. In short, you have little time to breathe. Since oxygen is the "food of life" no wonder you feel tired and everything seems too much for you.

Let your jaw drop open. Do not push it down, just let it drop! Now---more! Until you can get a small apple in your mouth. You should begin to feel a yawn coming that seems as though it will never end, one that closes your eyes and even makes them water a little bit.

Right! Perhaps you have discovered that when you yawn, you're also taking a deep breath and filling your lungs with oxygen. When the yawn ends, you feel relaxed all the way down to your stomach. Your lungs have expanded. The tension is releasing in your back.

In addition, you have relaxed your jaw, your mouth, and your tongue. Now you are no longer frowning. In fact, you should feel a bit of energy from the abundance of oxygen you drew into your system. It's amazing that such a small thing has such an effect, isn't it?

Try this often during the day. Stand in front of an open window if possible. A deep yawn before an important meeting or engagement will make you much more relaxed and refreshed.

146

PROPER BODY ALLIGNMENT

Here is another simple trick that will help you combat fatigue. Several times a day, stand against a wall, heels touching it, feet six inches apart. Now make your hips touch the wall, then your shoulders and finally your head. Stand tall. That pulled a bit, didn't it? Slowly walk away from the wall, still holding that posture.

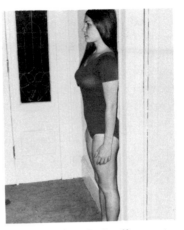

Proper body alignment

See what has happened? As you walked away from the wall, you became aware of proper body alignment. The sensation or feeling will stay with you for a while, even after you sit down, and help you maintain good posture.

After you walk away from the wall you may want to try an additional trick of body alignment. It will give a new sensation to your hands and arms. Take a deep breath, raise your arms from your sides to shoulder height and spread your fingers until you feel a slight pull on the fourth and fifth fingers. As your arms start to swing up, inhaling as you do so, you will enjoy a feeling of exaltation.

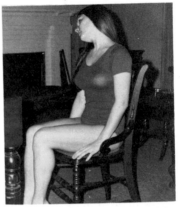

Head rotation relieves tension

Try these two tricks before you leave the house in the morning to get off to a good start. Also, try them at various times during the day or any time you have a spare minute. Relaxing, you see does not take alot of paraphernalia--- only you and a little know-how!

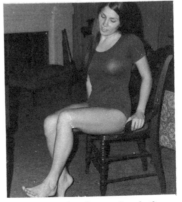

Wiggle stimulates circulation

147

RELIEF FOR ACHING EYES, NECK, AND SHOULDERS

Do your eyes burn, your neck and shoulders ache after sitting at a desk most of the day? Try this:

While seated in a chair, close your eyes and convince yourself that they are dropping forward in their sockets. You can see nothing at all, nothing but soft darkness. With your eyes still closed, let your head drop until your jaw is almost to your chest, and you feel the hinges of your jaw relax. Take a deep breath and begin to rotate your head. Just let it roll softly and slowly around the right, then back so it falls on the shoulders, and then to the left and forward. Did that hurt? Good! Feel the snap, crackle, pop? Take another deep breath and rotate the opposite way.

What has happened? You have begun to release that tension that was forming at the back of your neck. That tension not only hurt but made you feel that your vitality was at a low ebb.

Now here is a movement that will perform miracles in helping you release some of that shoulder tension. Take a deep breath, hold it and raise your right shoulder, roll it forward, up, back, and around in a complete circle. Exhale. This should be a slow rolling motion, not a jerky pull. Follow the same motion with the left shoulder.

Don't you feel better now? Remember, it is not the hard worker, but the relaxed worker that gets the job, who gets things done, who creates about her an atmosphere of confidence, who lives life to the very hilt and enjoys it.

YOUR BIG TOE

Few people realize the negative effect of aching and tense feet on the whole well-being of the body. The Chinese have a saying: "When the big toe is well, the body is well." This is the truth.

Here is a trick that could not be easier: just wiggle your toes especially the big one with your shoes on or off. That is right; move your toes up and down and from side to side. You can do this relaxing movement almost anywhere----at your desk, in a conference, at the movies, or in your car.

Here is another stimulator for tired feet and legs: try shaking your ankles for a few seconds to limber them. First wiggle one and then the other. You did not know that your ankles were that stiff, did you? Give them another quick shake.

There you have it. These are simple tricks that require five minutes at the most, sometimes one minute, sometimes only thirty seconds. A minute here and there between jobs, sitting at your desk, waiting for a bus, doing housework, can forestall fatigue, restore energy, and enable you to function at your peak.

Tension is our greatest enemy after middle age. Practice these tricks and you will soon be releasing tension and bringing on waves of relaxation. Isn't that worth five minutes?

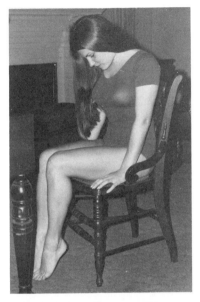

Practice a slow head rotation to relieve tension in your neck. Be sure to rotate both ways.

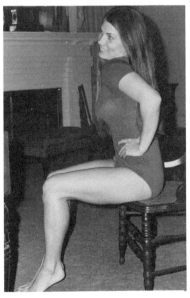

With hands on your hips try rotating your arm, forward, back, around. You should feel a release of tension in your shoulders.

PART
C
DIET & NUTRITION

INTRODUCTION TO DIET AND NUTRITION

The first article in this section, number seventeen, tells you how to evaluate your present nutritional status. Charts, tables, and guidelines are given for comparison purposes.

Losing body fat in a safe, sensible way is the subject for article eighteen. Fad diets are discussed. Rules are set down for selecting a well-balanced, low-calorie diet.

Facts about "health foods" are presented in the next article. After a thorough reading, you may realize that many of the special foods you are currently eating as *health* foods do not meet that criteria.

If you take "the pill," you will certainly want to read article twenty: "Facts Young Women Should Know About Oral Contraceptive Pills."Charts and tables in this chapter are particularly informative.

If you are an athlete who competes in an endurance-type sport, then your performance might be improved from a carbohydrate-rich diet. The twenty-first article will fill you in the why and how of this special dietary routine.

Bread has been praised. Bread has been condemned. In the final analysis, bread is deemed to be "King of the Basic Four." Find out why by reading article twenty-two.

When you are purchasing fresh fruits and vegetables, have you ever wished for some pointers on when to buy, how to store, and how to prepare? These questions will all be answered in "The ABC's of Fresh Fruits and Vegetables."

The last article in this section is "What Do You Feed a Hungry Girl?" This was written particularly for the coaches of teenage girls. Anyone, though, will benefit from the questions and answers presented here.

17

Determining Your Nutritional Status

DETERMINING YOUR NUTRITIONAL STATUS

To some people nutrition refers to the preparation and the service of tasty foods in an attractive manner. To others nutrition refers more to various agricultural practices used in the growth and development of healthy, marketable livestock. To yet others, it refers to cell processes and how cells receive their required nutrients. Actually, it includes all of these.

Nutrition is both a scientific discipline and a biological process. The scientific disciplines can be divided into the natural and social sciences. Nutrition belongs to the group of natural sciences or those that concern nature and the physical world. Natural sciences may be divided into those described as pure, such as mathmatics, physics, chemistry, and biology; and those described as applied, such as engineering, medicine, nutrition, agriculture, and geology. For this article, I shall define nutrition as the study of food and all the processes involved in its change from the time it is eaten until the wastes are excreted from the body.

This nutritional process may be successful, or it may be faulty in varying degrees at different points. The faults may result from the consumption of too little or too much food, the wrong kinds of food, or from a functional failure of one or more of the systems of the body. Thus, the integrated performance of your body's systems can be referred to as your nutritional status.

To make a thorough assessment of your nutritional status, you should view the task as a series of evaluations applied to the body as a whole,or to body areas, sensitive to nutritional measurements. Reduced to the simplest terms, such evaluations are the measure of an individual's body structure and how it feels, looks, and functions. For example, a woman in excellent nutritional status from birth can be expected to have (1) a well-developed skeleton with well-formed teeth and jaws,(2) a normal padding of fat over bones and muscles, and (3) a blood supply that carries adequate amounts of oxygen and nutrients to the cells. It is safe to predict most women with these basic characteristics of good nutritional status will be likely to display outward signs of vigor and health.

Determining your nutritional status requires sophisticated measuring techniques. Of course, these techniques are designed for use by specialists in various scientific fields. However, I shall briefly describe several of the methods and present standards for their use. Hopefully, you will be able to grasp how each type of evaluation contributes to a comprehensive assessment of your nutritional status.

Determining Your Nutritional Status

PHYSICAL EXAMINATION

The first step in the assessment of your nutritional status is a general physical examination. Physicians are aware that many nutritional deficiencies may be expressed by some of the following superficial signs and symptoms: stiff brittle hair; abnormally dry and rough skin; dry, dull, and lusterless eyes, with irritated lids; a deep red fissured tongue; spongy bleeding gums; lips that are swollen, chapped and cracked at the corners. All these symptoms may not always appear.

The second step in nutritional assessment should be the measurement of the body to perform its various functions, for example: color vision, vision in dim light, heart function, and work capacity.

Since these gross clinical signs and functions are easily observed, they are often used in making the initial tentative estimate of an individual's nutritional status.

However, they are general signs of ill health and do not necessarily indicate malnutrition. Malnutrition can be provoked by other factors such as infection, faulty digestion, absorption, utilization, or elimination.

The following diagram by a well-known British nutritionist Dr. H.M. Sinclair shows that your physical well-being is composed of many interrelated factors:

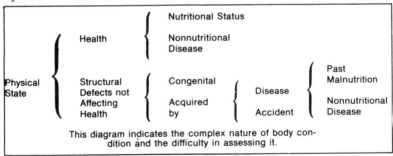

This diagram indicates the complex nature of body condition and the difficulty in assessing it.

HEIGHT AND WEIGHT

Desirable height and weight charts have been composed for men and women. Those averages are found in Table 1. Although it is difficult to state ideal weights, these tables present typical ranges of body weight among apparently healthy individuals according to height, age, sex, frame (size and weight of skeleton). However, the drawbacks of these charts are that they do not apply to many women, particularly athletes.

A better method of determining if you are overweight would be to use specific measurements of body fat.

155

TABLE 1
WEIGHTS FOR HEIGHTS OF MEN AND WOMEN

| | Weights for Men | | | Weights for Women | | |
| Height | Low | Median | High | Low | Median | High |
Inches	Pounds	Pounds	Pounds	Pounds	Pounds	Pounds
60	——	——	——	100	109	118
61	——	——	——	104	112	121
62	——	——	——	107	115	125
63	118	129	141	110	118	128
64	122	133	145	113	122	132
65	126	137	149	116	125	135
66	130	142	155	120	129	139
67	134	147	161	123	132	142
68	139	151	166	126	136	146
69	143	155	170	130	140	151
70	147	159	174	133	144	156
71	150	163	178	137	148	161
72	154	167	183	141	152	166
73	158	171	188	——	——	——
74	162	175	192	——	——	——
75	165	178	195	——	——	——

BODY FAT

Since overweight, or "overfat," is known to be unhealthy or un-desirable, a better estimate of general nutritional status would be the measurement of your percentage of body fat. A person is said to be o-bese (excessively overweight) when his body weight is 20% greater than his ideal weight. Several methods have been used to measure body fat, namely: X-rays, specific gravity, "potassium 40," and skin-fold thickness.

The easiest and most popular way of assessing the amount of body fat is measuring skinfold thickness. The thickness of a fold of skin in various areas of the body (triceps, abdomen, hips, thighs, etc.) is measured with skinfold calipers. Such thickness data can be translated into percentage of body fat. Although these data are not perfect, they do give a better indication of body fat than mere body weight and height data. Typically, the amount of body fat varies with sex and age. In general, it is greatest in infancy and diminishes in childhood and increases again during adolescence. Research indi-cates that girls and women generally have more body fat than do men and boys. An abnormally great or small amount of body fat is related to good or poor nutritional status, especially when compared with

156

body weight. Standards to aid in determining when the amount of body fat is abnormal are presented in Table 2. The table also indicates that the amount of fat in the triceps area varies throughout life.

Your own body fat can be estimated by the "pinch test." Pick up a pinch of skin from the back of an arm, midway between the elbow and shoulder (mid-triceps area). When you take your fingers away have a ruler handy so you can measure the distance between your fingers (to the nearest eighth of an inch). If the distance is more than 3/4 of an inch, the chances are you are overfat. Research has shown that the thickness of the skin in the mid-triceps area correlates fairly well with total body fat determined by more comprehensive measurements.

Most Americans have over 25% of their bodyweight in the form of fat. As you would suspect, athletes have a smaller percentage of fat than non-athletes. Table 3 shows the result of a recent study completed on Czechoslovakian athletes. You will notice that most of these athletes have a minimum of body fat.

An ideal amount of body fat for most female athletes would be from 10-12%. The average female interested in overall fitness should strive for 16-18% body fat.

COMPOSITION OF BLOOD AND URINE

A more precise but expensive way of assessing a person's nutritional status is to measure the nutrients circulating in the blood or being excreted in the urine. Such measurements actually reveal the tissue status of the nutrients and can be judged to be normal by comparison with data

TABLE 2. OBESITY STANDARDS FOR CAUCASIAN AMERICANS
Triceps Skinfold Thickness in Millimeters

Age (years)	Skinfold measurements	
	Males	Females
5	12	14
6	12	15
7	13	16
8	14	17
9	15	18
10	16	20
11	17	21
12	18	22
13	18	23
14	17	23
15	16	24
16	15	25
17	14	26
18	15	27
19	15	27
20	16	28
21	17	28
22	18	28
23	18	28
24	19	28
25	20	29
26	20	29
27	21	29
28	22	29
29	23	29
30-50	23	30

157

	Weight (lbs.)	% Body Fat
TABLE 3. BODY WEIGHT AND FATNESS OF 10 MEN AND 10 WOMEN CHAMPIONS IN DIFFERENT SPORTS		
MEN		
1. Gymnastics	148.7	4.5
2. Marathon runners	135.7	6.1
3. Weight lifting	170.3	6.2
4. Racing cycling	155.8	6.2
5. Tennis	138.2	7.3
6. Volleyball	174.7	7.5
7. Table tennis	128.7	9.2
8. Basketball	215.8	11.7
9. Ice hockey	148.1	14.8
10. Greco-Roman wrestling	227.0	19.0
WOMEN		
1. Gymnastics	122.3	8.3
2. Gymnastics	117.7	10.2
3. High jump	136.8	10.3
4. 10 m diving	110.0	12.4
5. Skiing 10 km	120.1	13.5
6. Swimming	153.6	13.8
7. Ice skating	128.3	15.3
8. Tennis	137.5	18.2
9. Table tennis	115.3	18.3
10. Shot put and discus	179.7	19.7

from healthy, well-nourished individuals of the same sex, age, physical development, and activity.

RECOMMENDED DIETARY STANDARDS

The nutrients required by women are widely distributed in common foods so that many   different diets provide adequate amounts of all the nutrients. For various reasons, however, some people restrict the number of different foods eaten. Some of these people are finicky eaters, some "health food" faddists, some poor people.

In order to help people eat the required nutrients in sufficient amounts, dietary standards have been established in many countries. These standards have been developed with the requirements of the people of each particular country in mind; the effects that cooking has on the nutritional value of the food; the digestibility and rate of absorption; and the expected variation in the nutrient quality of the food.

In Tables 4 and 5, there are listed several recommended dietary allowances established for young men and women in several countries. Recommendations have also been made for people of other ages.

You will note that all of these recommendatons are similar to the recommendations established for Americans by the National Research Council (see Tables 4 and 5).

FOOD HABITS AND DIET RECORDS

How does the fitness-minded woman know if she is eating correctly? Until she keeps a record of her daily eating habits, she probably does not realize how much of particular foods she consumes. In this respect, you are urged to "keep score" on the details of your diet. You need to know how much of which foods you consume for several days, both on week days and on weekend days. This will tell you which of your eating habits need improvement; the frequency of eating as well as the quality (nutrient content) and the quantity of the food consumed (see Tables 6 and 7).

The food scoreboard was developed according to the basic diet described by the Food and Nutrition Board of the National Research Council. This diet consists of two to four cups of milk or dairy products a day, two servings of meat, four or more servings of fruits and vegetables, and four or more servings in the bread group. By following this procedure you will be able to test the nutritional quality or adequacy of your diet.

Recent research shows that the average American consumes over 3,400 calories a day. Of these calories 45% comes from carbohydrates, 12% from proteins, and 43% from fat food sources. Nutrition and medical authorities are in agreement that Americans consume

Country	Sex	Age (years)	Weight (kg)	kcal	Protein (g)	Calcium (mg)	Iron (mg)	Vit. A activity (IU)	Thiamin (mg)	Riboflavin (mg)	Niacin equiv. (mg)	Ascorbic acid (mg)
U.S.A.	M	22	70	2,800	52	800	10	5,000	1.5	1.8	20	45
	F	22	58	2,000	46	800	18	4,000	1.1	1.4	14	45
FAO-WHO	M	25	65	3,200	46	400–500			1.3	1.8	21.1	
	F	25	65	2,300	39	400–500			0.9	1.3	15.2	
Australia	M	25	70	2,900	70	400–800	10	2,500	1.2	1.5	18	30
	F	25	58	2,100	58	400–800	10	2,500	0.8	1.1	14	30
Colombia	M	20–29	65	2,850	68	500	10	5,000	1.1	1.7	18.8	50
	F	20–29	55	1,900	60	500	15	5,000	0.8	1.1	12.5	50
Japan	M	26–29	56	3,000	70	600	10	2,000	1.5	1.5	15	65
	F	26–29	49	2,400	60	600	10	2,000	1.2	1.2	12	60
Norway	M	25	70	3,400	70	800	12	2,500	1.7	1.8	17	30
	F	25	60	2,500	60	800	12	2,500	1.3	1.5	13	30
Philippines	M	none specified	53	2,400	53	500		5,000	1.2	1.2		70
	F		46	1,800	46	500		5,000	0.9	0.9		70
West Germany	M	25	72	2,500	72	800	10	5,000	1.7	1.8	18	75
	F	25	60	2,200	60	800	12	5,000	1.5	1.8	14	75

TABLE 4. COMPARATIVE DIETARY STANDARDS OF SELECTED COUNTRIES AND U.N. AGENCIES

TABLE 5. FOOD AND NUTRITION BOARD, NATIONAL ACADEMY OF SCIENCES—NATIONAL RESEARCH COUNCIL RECOMMENDED DAILY DIETARY ALLOWANCES[a], REVISED 1973
Designed for the Maintenance of Good Nutrition of Practically all Healthy People in the U.S.A.

	(years) From	Up to	Wt (lbs)	Height (in)	Energy (kcal)	Protein (g)	Fat-Soluble Vitamins			Water-Soluble Vitamins								Minerals				
							Vitamin A Activity (IU)	Vita-min D Activity (IU)	Vita-min E Activity (IU)	Ascor-bic Acid (mg)	Fola-cin (µg)[2]	Nia-cin (mg)	Ribo-flavin (mg)	Thia-min (mg)	Vita-min B6 (mg)	Vita-min B12 (µg)	Cal-cium (mg)	Phos-phorus (mg)	Iodine (µg)	Iron (mg)	Mag-nesium (mg)	Zinc (mg)
INFANTS	0.0-0.5		14	24	kg × 117	kg × 2.2	1,400	400	4	35	50	5	0.4	0.3	0.3	0.3	360	240	35	10	60	3
	0.5-1.0		20	28	kg × 108	kg × 2.0	2,000	400	5	35	50	8	0.6	0.5	0.4	0.3	540	400	45	15	70	5
CHILDREN	1-3		28	34	1300	23	2,000	400	7	40	100	9	0.8	0.7	0.6	1.0	800	800	60	15	150	10
	4-6		44	44	1800	30	2,500	400	9	40	200	12	1.1	0.9	0.9	1.5	800	800	80	10	200	10
	7-10		66	54	2400	36	3,300	400	10	40	300	16	1.2	1.2	1.2	2.0	800	800	110	10	250	10
MALES	11-14		97	63	2800	44	5,000	400	12	45	400	18	1.5	1.4	1.6	3.0	1200	1200	130	18	350	15
	15-18		134	69	3000	54	5,000	400	15	45	400	20	1.8	1.5	1.8	3.0	1200	1200	150	18	400	15
	19-22		147	69	3000	52	5,000	400	15	45	400	20	1.8	1.5	2.0	3.0	800	800	140	10	350	15
	23-50		154	69	2700	56	5,000	—	15	45	400	18	1.6	1.4	2.0	3.0	800	800	130	10	350	15
	51+		154	69	2400	56	5,000	—	15	45	400	16	1.5	1.2	2.0	3.0	800	800	110	10	350	15
FEMALES	11-14		97	62	2400	44	4,000	400	10	45	400	16	1.3	1.2	1.6	3.0	1200	1200	115	18	300	15
	15-18		119	65	2100	48	4,000	400	11	45	400	14	1.4	1.1	2.0	3.0	1200	1200	115	18	300	15
	19-22		128	65	2100	46	4,000	400	12	45	400	14	1.4	1.1	2.0	3.0	800	800	100	18	300	15
	23-50		128	65	2000	46	4,000	—	12	45	400	13	1.2	1.0	2.0	3.0	800	800	100	18	300	15
	51+		128	65	1800	46	4,000	—	12	45	400	12	1.1	1.0	2.0	3.0	800	800	80	10	300	15
PREGNANCY	—	—	—	—	+300	+30	5,000	400	15	60	800	+2	+0.3	+0.3	2.5	4.0	1200	1200	125	18+[3]	450	20
LACTATION	—	—	—	—	+500	+20	6,000	400	15	60	600	+4	+0.5	+0.3	2.5	4.0	1200	1200	150	18	450	25

The allowances are intended to provide for individual variations among most normal persons as they live in the United States under usual environmental stresses. Diets should be based on a variety of common foods in order to provide other nutrients for which human requirements have been less well defined.

2. Microgram
3. This increased requirement cannot be met by ordinary diets; therefore, the use of supplemental iron is recommended.

too many calories. These calories are provided primarily by refined sugars and fat.

TABLE 6 ONE-DAY MEAL RECORD

1. Write down what you eat at each meal and between meals.
2. Look at the food group lists to identify each food (See Table 7).
3. Record food quantities in the food groups column.

EXAMPLE: BREAKFAST

	Milk Group	Meat Group	Fruits and Vegetables	Bread and Cereal	Additional Foods
½ cup orange juice			1		
1 egg		1			
2 slices of buttered toast				2	2
1 cup milk	1				

4. Transfer total scores to your "Food Scoreboard."

TYPICAL ONE-DAY MEAL RECORD

FOOD GROUPS

Meal	Milk Group (cups)	Meat Group (servings)	Fruits and Vegetables (servings)	Bread and Cereal (servings)	Additional Foods like fats, candy, desserts, soft drinks, snacks
Breakfast					
Mid-morning snack					
Lunch					
Afternoon snack					
Dinner					
Evening snack					
TOTALS					

Record other foods consumed throughout the day
in a similar manner on the "Typical One-Day Meal Record"
(Table 6) and then transfer these total amounts to the sample
"Food Scoreboard" which gives a breakdown of about 2,500 calories

TABLE 7.
REPRESENTATIVE FOOD LIST CLASSIFIED BY FOOD GROUPS: CALORIE VALUES IN SINGLE SERVINGS

Food	Weight or approximate measure	Calories	Food	Weight or approximate measure	Calories
Milk Group			**Fruit Group**		
Cheese, cheddar	1⅛ cube	115	Apple, raw	1 medium	70
Cheese, cottage, creamed	¼ cup	65	Apricots, dried, stewed	½ cup	135
Cream, coffee	1 tbsp	30	Banana, raw	1 medium	100
Milk, fluid, skim (buttermilk)	1 cup	90	Cantaloupe	½ melon	60
Milk fluid, whole	1 cup	160	Grapefruit	½ medium	45
Meat Group			Orange	1 medium	65
Beans, dry, canned	¾ cup	233	Orange juice, fresh	½ cup (small glass)	55
Beef, pot roast	3 oz.	245	Peaches, canned	½ cup with syrup	100
Chicken	½ breast—with bone	155	Pineapple juice, canned	½ cup (small glass)	68
Egg	1 medium	80	Prunes, dried, cooked	5 with juice	160
Frankfurter	1 medium	170	Strawberries, raw	½ cup, capped	30
Haddock	1 fillet	140	**Bread-cereal Group**		
Ham, boiled	2 oz.	135	Bread, white, enriched	1 slice	70
Liver, beef	2 oz.	130	Cornflakes, fortified	1½ cup	133
Peanut butter	2 tbsp	190	Macaroni, enriched, cooked	¾ cup	115
Pork chop	1 chop	260	Oatmeal, cooked	⅔ cup	87
Salmon, canned	½ cup	120	Rice, cooked	¾ cup	140
Sausage, bologna	2 slices	173	**Fats Group**		
Vegetable Group			Bacon, crisp	2 slices	90
Beans, snap, green	½ cup	15	Butter or fortified margarine	1 tbsp	100
Broccoli	½ cup	20	Oils, salad or cooking	1 tbsp	125
Cabbage, shredded, raw	½ cup	10	**Sweets Group**		
Carrots, diced	½ cup	23	Beverages, cola type	6 oz.	75
Corn, canned	½ cup	85	Sugar, granulated	1 tbsp	40
Lettuce leaves	2 large or 4 small	10			
Peas, green	½ cup	58			
Potato, white	1 medium	90			
Spinach	½ cup	20			
Squash, winter	½ cup	65			
Sweet potato	1 medium	155			
Tomato juice, canned	½ cup (small glass)	23			

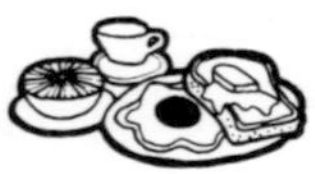

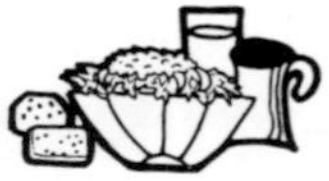

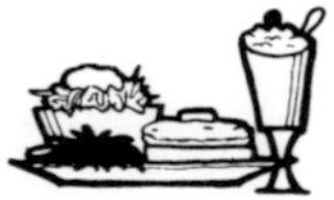

Determining Your Nutritional Status

FOOD SCOREBOARD (approximately 2,500 calories)

Recommended Food	Goal	Score
Milk	3 cups	_____
Meat	5 servings	_____
Fruit	6 servings	_____
Vegetables	2 servings	_____
Bread	4 servings	_____
Other	2 teaspoons oil	_____
	2 desserts	_____

Take a look at your score.
You may find you have been leaving out important foods
If so , you may find you have too many "empty calories"
such as carbonated beverages and candy

Foods to Add	Foods to Cut Down On
1._____	1. _____
2. _____	2. _____
3. _____	3. _____

Americans consume many pastries and other desserts, foods fried in fat, and a lot of beef. The average American eats over 100 grams of protein each day, primarily in the form of meat and dairy products. Although these foods contain high-quality protein, amounts eaten in excess of body needs are converted to fat. Furthermore, they contain an appreciable amount of fat which is the most concentrated form of energy in the diet.

Authorities also recommend that the fat content of the American diet should be reduced by 30%. The optimum diet for health should look like this as far as proportions are concerned:

	Fat	Protein	Carbohydrate
Average American Diet	43%	12%	45%
Optimum Diet for Health	30%	12%	58%

Using these guidelines, I have developed diets for two energy levels. One diet provides 2,500 calories a day; the other provides

163

TABLE 8
TOTAL SERVINGS OF FOODS IN DAILY MEAL SCHEDULES

Approximate Calories	Whole Milk	Meat or Equivalent	Fruit	Veg.	Bread	Other
2500	3 cups	5 ounces	6 ser.	2 ser.	8 ser. 4 with jelly	2 desserts 2 teaspoon oil
3750	4½ cups	7½ ounces	9 ser.	3 ser.	12 ser. 6 with jelly	3 desserts 3 teaspoon oil
5000	6 cups	10 ounces	12 ser.	4 ser.	16 ser. 8 with jelly	4 desserts 4 teaspoon oil

TABLE 9
APPROXIMATE NUTRIENT CONTENT OF DAILY MEAL SCHEDULE

	FAT		PROTEIN		CARBOHYDRATE	
Approximate Calories	Grams	% Total Calories	Grams	% Total Calories	Grams	% Total Calories
2500	70	28	79	13	374	59
3750	105	28	118	13	561	59
5000	140	28	158	13	748	59

3,750 calories a day. They are especially geared for female athletes. You will find these diets put the emphasis on carbohydrates, which are most efficiently used by the body for energy production. The diets are described by listing the appropriate amounts of the food groups, as well as their nutrient content (see Tables 8 and 9).

You will notice that the nutrient content of these daily schedules is almost the same as the "Optimum Diet for Health." I have added an extra percentage point for the athlete in protein and carbohydrate foods and deducted two from the fat sources. I believe this will benefit the athlete's performance.

The daily meal schedules were developed for two energy levels: 2,500 and 3,750 calories. From these two diets, you should be able to plan your own special diet. For example, a 135-pound golfer might require 2,500 calories a day, as well as the 110-pound gymnist. On the other hand, a female basketball player or long-distance swimmer might require 3,750.

With this article's advice and charts, you should be able to make your nutritional status a good one.

Body Fat:
To Have and To Hold...
OR...To Lose

18

BODY FAT
To Have and To Hold---OR---To Lose

Tired of looking and feeling flabby? This article presents solid and sensible information on how to lose that flab.

Just answer these questions:

1. Does your stomach bulge even when you pull it in?
2. Are there " handles" on the outside of your thighs?
3. Do you have pudgy arms?
4. Is your hip measurement more than three inches larger than your bust measurement?
5. Do you have a "wandering" waistline or difficulty in pinpointing exactly where it is?
6. Do you have saggy breasts?

Statistics show that over half the women in the United States have one or more of these problems. Authorities agree that most Americans are too fat and prone toward obesity.

"But how," you say, "can I lose this awful fat? I have tried diet after diet, after diet with no permanent results."

First, chin up. IT CAN BE DONE. But, it takes proper know-how----plus discipline and patience.

Calories and balance are the key words. There is no other healthy way to treat, or more accurately put, to control obesity. If you want to reduce body fat, keep it off, and not harm yourself in the process, you must practice self-discipline. It is this self-discipline that is needed to adhere to a low-calorie, balanced diet. This requires both motivation and patience.

You must not waver in your determination to change your style of life and eating habits. Once you have made the change, you must abide by the new regimen no matter how great the temptation is to stray from this straight and narrow path.

These are the harsh, plain realities. Perhaps because they are so simple and stark, obesity remains the biggest health problem in America today.

Although there are many fine points involved in the effective application of the simple rules of caloric restriction and nutritional balance, they are all that sound medical and nutritional science has to offer for the management of obesity at this time. No wonder so many people seek a way out of this difficult-to-accept reality and turn to some "magic" diet formula instead.

To help clear the air, let's examine and analyze some recent fad diets.

166

FAD DIETS

All diets, balanced or unbalanced, will produce weight loss (but not necessarily fat loss) if the total calories they provide in twenty-four hours is less than your caloric requirement for weight maintenance. Certainly weight loss will appear to be somewhat faster on some diets than on others. But no diet will result in loss of fat if it ignors the principle of the conservation of energy and the first law of thermodynamics by not providing for significant caloric restriction.

Probably the most misleading type of fad diet is derived from the school of thought that permits unlimited consumption of certain high-protein foods. Examples are the "Calories Don't Count Diet" which adds safflower oil to unlimited proteins and fat with very little carbohydrates; the "All the Meat You Want Diet;" and the "Doctor's Quick Weight Loss Diet" which allows unlimited amounts of certain meat, fish, eggs, and cheeses and requires drinking at least eight glasses of water a day.

The life span of each of these diets is brief because it takes at most a few days or weeks for the people misled into following them to discover they cannot continue this regimen. The reason for failure of these diets is simple enough: *they run counter to the best principles of balance, minimal change, and the teaching of good dietary habits for permanent control.*

After a short time on one of these diets, you are only able to force down a limited amount of calories. As a result, you frequently do lose weight simply because you become bored with eating the same foods and eat less.

Another type of fad diet may require some caloric restriction but demands either a sharp reduction of carbohydrate intake or no carbohydrates at all. An example of this is the "Drinking Man's Diet" which substitutes alcohol for carbohydrates. Alcohol contains no nutrients but many calories.

Other diets of this type have been cloaked in a mantle of respectability by such names as the "Mayo Diet"—a name that has been applied over the years to a number of diets, none of which had the slightest connection with this reknowned clinic. The latest in diets which steal their names from respectable institutions is the "Air Force Diet" which has been emphatically disowned by the Air Force.

The most famous of the low-carbohydrate diets is "Dr. Atkin's Diet." In this diet the carbohydrates are reduced to sixty grams or less while fat and protein are usually unlimited. The "scientific" explanation offered for this diet's alleged effectiveness is: a fat person's carbohydrate is rapidly converted to fat tissue, rather than being used for energy, whereas calories from fat and protein are burned up in the metabolic process and are not stored as body fat. *This is simply not true.*

What does appear to be true to some extent is that excess calories from whatever source are less readily utilized and more readily stored in a fat person. The intially greater weight loss that results from a low-carbohydrate diet (as compared to a balanced one with the same number of calories) is actually due to loss of body water, not body fat. Ignorance of this scientifically proven fact has probably led to more confusion in the dietary treatment of obesity than any other single fact.

To understand this concept, a differentation must be made between fat loss and scale-weight loss. The scale measures total weight only and cannot distinguish fat loss from water loss or loss of vital lean tissue. A diet that contains carbohydrates, but is well below your caloric requirements, will produce a reduction in scale weight that will parellel fat loss for only a few weeks. Then, although your body fat continues to decrease, retention of water will set in and mask or counter balance the fat loss. If a diet contains little or no carbohydrates, this disturbing phenomenon does not occur.

Yet, carbohydrate must be furnished in a diet, despite this disadvantage for a number of important reasons. First of all, if lifetime calorie control is to be acceptable, the diet must have some palatability and appeal. Much of variety and taste in foods is supplied by carbohydrates. In addition, carbohydrates are essential nutrients. Your body has a specific need for carbohydrates as a source of energy for the brain as well as other specialized functions. The Food and Nutrition Board of the National Research Council has said that a normal adult requires approximately 500 carbohydrate calories a day.

The greatest "crash" diet of all time is that of total fasting. Here you are given only liquids and, of course, no protein. Adequate protein intake is a basic requirement for health. A reducing diet, just like a normal diet, must contain sufficient protein to maintain the body structure. If this is not furnished in the reducing diet, the need will be filled by a breakdown in the body's lean, non-fat, protein tissue. Most of this will come from muscle, and some of it from organ tissue. Naturally, this is physiologically undesirable.

OVER-THE-COUNTER REDUCING FADS

Other examples of economic frauds are over-the-counter drugs and reducing aids which include candy, gum, tablets, capsules, and time-release pills. These so-called diet pills offer "a wonderful kind of plan to get rid of 5, 10, 25, or more pounds of unsightly fat. Not by suffering thru starvation dieting hunger . . . not by sticking to boring diets . . . not by extra tiring exercises." These products, according to their manufacturer, are for people who "love to eat."

The package of reducing pills may mention a plan as well as supply you with the pills. It will say "Product X with a diet plan." These booklets which are sometimes as long as forty-two pages, advise you that the only way to lose weight is to eat less. Eating less means being on a diet; and in fact, these plans advise a highly restricted caloric diet.

Purchasers of these "reducing aids" are paying a high price, and at best, are buying a diet. This same type of diet is available in most women's magazines.

The sales of appetite control products, according to the November 1975 *Chain Store/Drug Edition,* is up 45%. The sale of these products expands by 20% per year. Sales this year are expected to be ninety million dollars. These products are among the fastest growing sellers in drugstores today.

You need to know what is contained in these fraudulent and expensive products. The Food and Drug Administration's Over-the-Counter Panel of Miscellaneous Internal Drug Products has divided them into three categories:

1. Those containing a combination of benzocaine, methylcellose, and sucrose (sold as mints, gum, candy).

2. Those containing a combination of phenylpropanolamine (PPA) and caffeine (most of these are sold as diet tablets).

3. Those containing alginic acid, sodium carboxymethylcellulose, and sodium bicarbonate (these are sold as candy and wafers).

One of the drugs is simply a candy with vitamins. All the products claim to control appetite and in that way induce weight loss.

Let us briefly consider these products. The diuretics sold over-the-counter are very weak and produce only a slight loss of water.

They produce no loss of fat at all. There have been no conclusive studies about the side effects of these drugs, but it is safe to say that if they produced dramatic weight loss, they would do it by dehydration which is dangerous if a person has heart, liver, or kidney disease. In short, these drugs should not be used for the treatment of obesity.

Some of these drugs contain small amounts of propanaoamine. Propanaoamine is an amphetamine-like drug with all the advantages and disadvantages of amphetamines. Amphetamines are not recommended because they produce only brief appetite suppression; and, worse yet, they are addicting. The same can be said for propanaoamine. In a well-controlled study that was run for two years, propanaoamine has not been shown to cause any weight loss.

Other diet pills contain an ingredient that produces bulk in the stomach and consequently gives a feeling of fullness. No long term studies have been made of these products, but a person could produce the same effect by eating a lot of carrots.

Benzocaine is supposed to anaesthetize the taste buds so that food does not taste good. Again, there is no scientific evidence to support this product's claim that it helped produce weight loss. In fact, there is no scientific evidence that any of these "magic potions" produce sustained weight loss.

Dr. James Ramey, Clinical Professor of Medicine at George Washington Medical School, states flatly that all the over-the-counter appetite/weight loss control claims are nonsense and lies. He says, "The laws of thermodynamics hold for humans; matter is neither created or destroyed. The only way to lose weight is to eat fewer calories than the body burns. None of the over-the-counter products aid dieting in the long run. Until they are shown to be effective, they should be withdrawn from the market."

The simple truth is: buying pills will help you lose money but not fat. The most these products can do is serve as a psychological crutch to help a dieter eat less. Although the pharmaceutical industry has tried to develop a satisfactory weight reduction drug, none has been developed. A person cannot lose fat by consuming a capsule, a candy, a pill.

Before getting to the nutritionally balanced diet that can actually help you lose weight, let us look at some factors that influence storing and losing of body fat.

FACTORS THAT INFLUENCE BODY FAT

1. Basal metabolic rate. This refers to the rate at which your body uses energy to maintain itself during a state of complete rest. Your body's regulator for basal metabolic rate is thyroxin, a hormone secreted by the thyroid gland. If there is a deficiency in the amount produced, a lower metabolic rate will result, thus reducing the total caloric requirement. Conversely, an overproduction of thyroxin will increase metabolic activity and caloric expenditure. Malfunctioning of the thyroid and other glands, however, appears to play only a minor role in the problem of overweight. In a study of 275 obese people, less than 3% had a glandular disorder that was to blame for their obesity.

2. Efficiency of the digestive system. There is a definite variation in the digestive systems of individuals. They differ in their ability to break down the energy component of food. A woman with an efficient system is able to supply the body with more calories from the same amount of food than a woman with an inefficient system. This creates the need for greater expenditure of energy through activity or a lower intake for an equal amount of work. Digestive efficiency, though, is difficult to determine without extensive medical tests.

3. Appetite regulating system. Generally speaking, appetite is thought to be controlled by a part of the brain called the hypothalmus. The hypothalmus is sensitive to the amount of sugar in the blood. Low sugar levels stimulate the appetite. Some authorities think the appetite of an obese person is more attuned to the sight, smell, and taste of food than the appetite of the non-obese person.

4. Fat tissue cell size. The fat cells in obesity are often increased in number as well as size. This is particularly true if obesity began in childhood or is extreme. Thus, a greater number of fat cells means an increased cell mass, even when individual cells are normal in content. If an obese woman mobilized fat from these normal-sized but more numerous fat cells, she would still have a relatively large mass of fat cells containing relatively little fat. This constitutes a barrier to weight reduction because, while fat cells can be created, they cannot be destroyed.

5. Heredity and environment. Studies have shown that three out of four obese people come from families with a history of obesity. Whether this tendency toward obesity is caused by hereditary factors or acquired by family eating habits has not been clearly determined.

Although heredity is a possible factor, a more likely cause seems to be the overeating habit from family and cultural attitudes. In some families preparing and serving an array of attractive, high-calorie meals is considered an expression of love rather than a means of providing needed nourishment for the body. Another cultural attitude that leads to overeating is the adage: the plate must be cleaned. Overeating habits developed from attitudes and patterns that were instilled in childhood are difficult to correct.

6. Emotional overeating. Emotional and personality factors are often a part of overeating. When lonely, frustrated, or unhappy, some people turn to food for pyschological release. In many respects, overeating is similar to addiction to alcohol, smoking, or drugs. This tendency is often reinforced by family customs of using food as a "reward" for good behavior or as a consolation during difficult times.

7. Water retention. In some people, especially women, there is a tendency to retain excessive water. This is distressing for those working toward weight control. The condition is called "edema" or bloating, and has nothing to do with calorie intake or expenditure. Edema in women quite often begins just before the menstrual period and continues throughout the period. During such times, the elimination of certain foods such as salt, pickles, salted butter, salted or cured fish and meats, and crackers can be helpful. For those with special water retention problems, a variety of diuretics (drugs that increase urinal production) may be helpful. These drugs should be prescribed by a physician.

NUTRITIONAL REQUIREMENTS FOR A BALANCED DIET

It should be obvious that fat loss by dieting can be accomplished by caloric reduction. The best way to restrict your food is by actually counting calories. Two precautions must be taken, however. First, an adequate food calorie chart or predetermined total calorie meal plan should be used; and second, the diet must meet the nutritional requirements of the body.

The three major classes of nutrients that your body needs are carbohydrates, proteins, and fats. Other nutrients include vitamins and minerals.

The food necessary to supply these nutrients for the repair, energy, and growth needs of the body can be broken into four groups:

Meat Group. Meat, fish, cheese, beans, dried peas, eggs, nuts, and poultry are included in this group. These foods are high in protein and contain ample amounts of fat. Daily intake should include two or more servings, preferably with each meal supplying some protein from these sources.

Milk Group. Adults do not outgrow their need for dairy products (at least two servings a day are needed). This group includes whole and skimmed milk, buttermilk, yogurt, cottage cheese, ice cream, and cheese. Protein, fat, and calcium are all found in dairy products.

Fruit and Vegetable Group. There should be three or four servings from this group a day, with both green and yellow fruits and vegetables included. Fruits and vegetables are an excellent source of carbohydrates, vitamins, and minerals.

Bread and Cereal Group. This group includes enriched or whole grain breads and cereals. There should be three to four servings included a day. The primary contribution of this group is to carbohydrate energy, but it also contains protein, vitamins, and minerals.

The chart, at the end of the article, that is based on selections from the Four Basic Food Groups, should be useful to all dieters. With this chart, you will find guidelines for 1,200 and 1,500 calorie diets.

FINAL CONSIDERATIONS

Recent studies show that over 75% of all Americans are prone to overweight. As a result, many people die prematurely. Most women reduce for the wrong reasons—usually for looks. They fail to realize that obesity is a major health hazard. If all deaths from cancer were eliminated, two years would be added to the average life span. If all deaths related obesity were removed, the life span would jump seven years. An astonishing fact!

The average moderately active woman needs approximately fifteen calories per pound of body weight per day to maintain her present body weight. To calculate your energy requirements multiply your weight by fifteen.

The American Medical Association recommends a weight loss of NO MORE than two pounds of body fat per week without the supervision of a physician. Beside the possible injurious side-effects of such excess weight loss, the loss of more than two pounds a week also results in the loss of muscle tissue.

There is no scientific evidence to show that weight control programs based on water loss (such as sauna or steam baths) are of value in a fat-reducing program. When a person drinks liquid after such a weight loss, the lost weight is regained.

The President's Council on Physical Fitness and Sports warns of the danger associated with a quick weight loss induced by loss of water. The warning reads, "Do not wear rubberized or plastic clothing while exercising to increase sweating as this will not cause permanent loss of body weight and can be harmful to your health. Rubberized or plastic clothing can cause body temperature to rise to a dangerous level because it does not give the sweat a chance to evaporate. When sweat cannot evaporate, body temperature increases, causing more sweating and leading to excessive dehydration and salt loss.

Remember----your excess body fat can be lost. But it takes know-how----discipline----patience.

I have given you the KNOW-HOW. You must supply the DISCIPLINE and PATIENCE. Good luck!

DIETARY GUIDELINES FOR LOSING FAT

(Sample Diets)

Food	For 1,200 Calories Daily	For 1,500 Calories Daily	Notes
Meat Group	3 small servings (or a total of 7 ounces cooked weight)	3 small servings (or a total of 7 ounces cooked weight)	Choose lean, well-trimmed meats: beef, veal, lamb, pork. Poultry and fish should have skin removed. One egg can be substituted for 1 serving of meat.
Milk Group	2 cups fortified skim milk	2 cups whole milk	Two cups milk means two 8-ounce measuring cups.
Fruits and Vegetables	4 servings	4 servings	One fruit serving = 1 medium fruit, 2 small fruits (i.e., apricots), 1/2 banana, 1/4 cantaloupe, 10-12 grapes or cherries, 1 cup fresh berries or 1/2 cup fresh, canned or frozen unsweetened fruit or fruit juice. Include one citrus fruit or other good source of vitamin C daily.

One vegetable serving = 1/2 cup cooked or 1 cup raw leafy vegetable. Include one dark green or deep-yellow vegetable or other good source of vitamin A at least every other day. |
| Bread and Cereal Group | 4 servings | 5 servings | One serving = 1 slice bread; 1 small dinner roll; 1/2 cup cooked cereal, noodles, macaroni, spaghetti, rice, cornmeal; 1 ounce (about 1 cup) ready-to-eat unsweetened iron-fortified cereal. |
| Other Foods | 1 serving | 3 servings | One serving = 1 teaspoon butter, margarine, or oil; 6 nuts; 2 teaspoons salad dressing; or 35 calories or less of another food. |

Note: Unless you are dieting under a doctor's supervision, don't go below 1,000 calories a day.

175

19

Sense and Nonsense about "Health Foods"

SENSE AND NONSENSE ABOUT "HEALTH FOODS"

Did you have brewer's yeast in your orange juice this morning? Have you had your wheat germ oil today? And what about vitamin C pills, high-protein tablets, and yogurt? Can forgetting to take any of these products each day be a serious detriment to your maximum athletic performance? Also, can eating enriched white bread and non-organic fruits and vegetables result in a multitude of bad consequences for that body of yours?

These are only a few of the confusing recommendations for vim and vigor that come from "health food" faddists. But, how true are beliefs that these foods will actually improve your health and performance?

Observations and interviews conducted at the Munich Olympics lead me to estimate that almost 50% of the American competitiors consumed some type of "health food" during their training. For example, Phil Grippaldi of the U.S. weightlifting team took seven different vitamin pills at each meal plus a liver-protein supplement. The late Steve Prefontaine, the U.S. record holder in the 3,000 and 5,000 meter runs, started each day with a breakfast drink that included brewer's yeast and wheat germ oil. Olympic champion Mark Spitz frequently ate yogurt to settle his stomach. These were not the only athletes dependent, to a greater or lesser extent, upon "health foods."

Should you, too, be consuming these foods? Will they provide you with more energy? Greater strength? Improve your athletic ability? Generally make you healthier? Before answering these questions, let us take a look at what these "health foods" are, and what they claim to do.

POPULAR "HEALTH FOODS"

Organically Grown Foods

"Organically grown" means that food has not been subjected to pesticides or artificial (chemical) fertilizers and has been grown in soil whose humus content has been increased by the addition of organic matter. Food faddists claim that organically grown foods are superior to other foods because they:(1) do not have poisonous residues that are found in chemically produced foods,(2) reduce pollution, (3) contain no harmful food additives,(4) taste better and are more nutritious.

The fact is, though, that nutrition scientists cannot accept the argument that agricultural chemicals are a threat to the safety of our food supply. Recently Dr. Hilda White of Northwestern University said that if modern agricultural technology were to be discarded in favor of organic farming, the worldwide problems of hunger, malnutrition, and famine would be multiplied immeasurably. Without pesticides and food additives, few families could afford adequate diets.

Wheat Germ

Wheat germ is the most nutritous part of the wheat plant. It is often destroyed during the milling of wheat flour. It is a rich source of B vitamins, protein, and vitamin E and can be eaten in a number of ways. When toasted, wheat germ becomes a tasty cereal with a nut-like flavor. When used as oil, it can be eaten in salads; or some athletes drink the oil straight from the bottle. The problem with such foods is that unmilled whole grains and oils easily turn rancid and moldy if they are not refrigerated. For this reason, they must be eaten relatively soon after processing.

Some people claim that wheat germ can prevent aging, muscular dystrophy, heart disease, as well as make you sexually potent. Also, many athletes believe that wheat germ increases their strength and endurance. The fact is, though, none of these claims that wheat germ is a unique supplier of some essential therapeutic ingredients have been substantiated. Wheat germ is NOT an essential food; it is NOT unique or magic. Enriched flour, fruits, vegetables, meat dairy products, and many other foods supply the same nutrients found in wheat germ.

Brewer's Yeast

Brewer's yeast is a bitter, yellow powder which is related to a variety of yeast that is a by-product of beer brewing. Thus, it is actually misnamed "brewer's yeast." It does however, contain large amounts of B vitamins, amino acids, and minerals. Supplementing the diet with dried brewer's yeast might be useful if you are deficient in protein and B vitamins; but eating brewer's yeast is not the most efficient or the most appetizing way to obtain these nutrients. Besides, only vitamins obtainable by a prescription contain B vitamins in high enough doses to be therapeutically valuable.

Honey

Food faddists have long promoted honey as a sweet that is better tolerated than other sugars. This is not true! Honey contains two types of sugar, glucose and fructose. These are simple sugars that are yielded in the digestion of table sugars or sucrose. Both honey and table sugar are quickly digested, and their glucose is available to the body for use. Honey is not significantly superior to other common sweets. It is an expensive way to get "empty calories" since honey contains little or no minerals.

Taken in large quanities, honey can produce several detrimental effects on athletes. Excess amounts of honey, glucose, dextrose, cubes of sugar, or other similar sweets tend to draw fluid from other parts of the body into the digestional tract. This shift in fluids may add to the problem of dehydration in endurance-type sports, where sweat loss can affect performance.

The body may also rebel if the sugar intake is too high. A concentrated sugar solution may cause distention in the stomach, and evacuation mechanisms may be impaired. Problems such as cramps, nausea, and diarrhea can occur. Therefore, no more than 50 grams of sugar (3 rounded teaspoons) in a liquid should be taken during any one-hour lapse. Even then, these foods do not seem to improve performance in short-term events.

Certified Raw Milk

While certified raw milk may contain somewhat larger amounts of certain nutrients than regular homogenized and pasteurized milk, it is more expensive and dangerous. "Health food" devotees point out that pasteurization destroys most of the beneficial hormones, enzymes, steroids, and a larger part of the fat and water soluble vitamins in milk.

Although it is true that pasteurization destroys some nutrients in milk, the value of pasteurization to health was proven long ago. To safely market unpasteurized milk, which is free from harmful bacteria, would necessitate impeccable hygiene and constant supervison of cows, equipment, and employees. The greater ease in processing pasteurized milk as well as safer finished product, far outweighs the advantage of supplying a few more nutrients. Those lost nutrients can easily be obtained from other foods.

Yogurt

Yogurt is a fermented milk product. Like all milk products, it is an excellent source of protein and calcium. Since most supermarkets have been carrying yogurt since the early 1960's, only very esoteric forms are sold in "health food" stores. Their prices are usually double those for grocery store yogurt. Yogurt is supposed to aid the digestion by regulating the balance of intestinal bacteria. However, chemical analyses have shown that it does not contain any miracle producing ingredient. Yogurt has the same food value as buttermilk, which is considerably less expensive.

Desiccated Liver

Desiccated liver, in pill or powder form, is a good source of vitamin B-12. Vitamin B-12 is vital for protection against pernicious anemia, which results in weakness and loss of energy and stamina. Faddists reason that if desiccated liver can keep you from getting weak and rundown from anemia, it would also aid in developing stamina. Numerous athletes have been known to take desiccated liver tablets by the handful, even over 100 a day.

Actually pernicious anemia is a very rare condition occuring in those who eat a vegetarian diet, or who have had their stomach totally removed, or those who have a genetic depot and cannot absorb the vitamin B-12 in their diet. Desiccated liver probably would not help the latter group because they could not absorb the vitamin B-12 in it. Intramuscular injections of this vitamin or a preparation to improve absorption, is usually given.

Protein Supplements

Pills and powders containing various kinds of proteins have been favorite supplements for athletes for years. Here are some examples of foods from which protein supplements are derived: skimmed milk powder, powdered liver, yeast, egg whites, preparations from beef spleen, heart, kidneys, pancreas, soya lecithin, calcium caseinate, pectin, and red bone marrow.

Numerous athletes and coaches assume that vigorous training increases the need for dietary protein. There is little scientific evidence to support this belief. In fact, carbohydrates and fats are preferred sources of energy for the body, not proteins! The National Research Council recommends that both men and women consume, on a daily basis, 0.8 grams of protein per kilogram (2.2 pounds) of bodyweight. This is more than enough protein to supply the tissue needs of an athlete.

Natural Vitamin and Mineral Supplements

The walls of most "health food" stores are lined with bottles of vitamin and mineral pills. The vitamins and minerals can be purchased both individually (vitamin A, D, B-6, and thiamin) or in multiple combinations. They come in all shapes, sizes, and quanities. They are guaranteed to cure almost anything from the common cold to rheumatism.

Faddists are quick to promote the vitamins from natural sources as opposed to the vitamins that are produced synthetically. Basically there is no difference between natural and synthetic vitamins, except for the higher cost of the natural ones.

Do athletes really need these vitamin and mineral supplements? The simple truth is: any well-balanced diet supplies all the essential nutrients that most athletes need during training. The one exception is during hot and humid weather when particular attention should be paid to replacing sodium chloride (salt) in the tissues. This can be done by frequently drinking salt water (0.1-0.2 percent concentration) or taking slow-release sodium chloride tablets before, during, and after training.

Vitamin requirements are not increased before or during strenuous exercise; and it is impossible to supercharge the tissues. Furthermore, with fat-soluable vitamins (A, D, E, and K) there is a danger of an overdose, since they can be stored in the body. The use of vitamin and mineral pills without a specific deficiency represents nothing more than the use of expensive placebos.

CONCLUSION

Why are athletes particularly susceptible to "health food" propaganda? Perhaps it is because their tremendous drive and motivation to compete and win makes them curious about any product that supposedly will improve their performance.

Once an athlete begins to approach the maximum achievement possible for an event, she often begins a desperate search for something new to add to her training program that will give her an edge over her competition. "Health foods" seem to offer a magic solution.

It is possible that the psychological benefit derived from consuming supplements, alleged to have remarkable powers, could make the difference in championship competition. Often psychological rather than physiological factors determine limits of performance. But, if this is the only contribution "health foods" are making, can such a nutritional program be justified in terms of costs and possible health hazzards? I think not.

Actually the term "health food" is a misnomer says the American Medical Association. They say the health of an individual is the result of many factors. Just one of these factors is food. The body does not require any particular food. It uses some fifty nutrients in varying amounts. None of these nutrients is considered a "health" nutrient; but, by definition, any nutrient that's required for human nutrition is essential to life and health even though some are needed in very small amounts. This is why I find it difficult to take the words "health foods" out of quotes.

What can you do to make sure you are properly nourished? You can begin by consuming a well-balanced diet each day. A well-balanced diet includes items from the Four Basic Food Groups: 1) two or more servings from the meat group, 2) at least two cups of milk or dairy products, 3) four or more servings of fruits and vegetables, and 4) four more more servings of bread and cereal.

If you eat these foods in moderation and diversity, avoid tension and stress, get plenty of exercise and enough rest; then, most illnesses of deficiency or of oversufficiency can be avoided. As for other ills, many have nothing to do with diet, despite the claims of "health food" evangelists.

In summary, the products sold in "health food" stores will not provide you with greater strength, energy, athletic ability, health, or you name it. At least not more than the products sold at your local supermarket. Stick to a well-balanced diet and try to realize that victory in the arena is more dependent on genetic factors and hard training than food. But, whatever you do, do not be misled by the claims of "health foods."

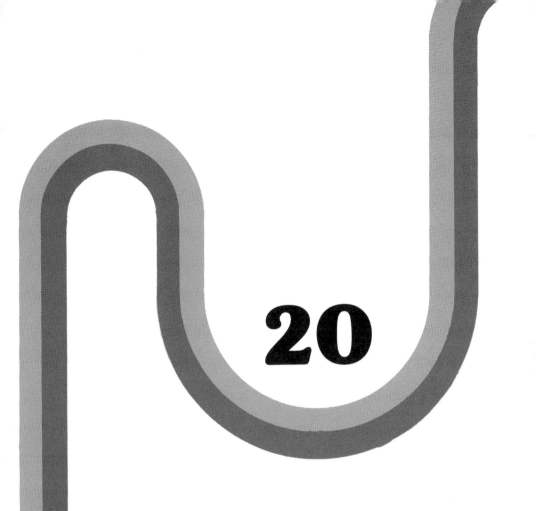

20

**Facts Young Women
Should Know about
Oral Contraceptive Pills**

FACTS YOUNG WOMEN SHOULD KNOW ABOUT
ORAL CONTRACEPTIVE PILLS

"**D**octor, should I take the pill?"

This question is asked thousands of times each day by women. Why? Because the search for a sure-fire method of birth control is as old as Adam's fig leaf and Eve's apple. Also, the expanding population is currently one of our most serious problems.

The number of women taking oral contraceptives, or simply "the pill," is a rather closely guarded secret. Some authorities estimate that it is well over ten million. If this figure is correct, then approximately 20% of the fifty million fertile women in the United States take "the pill." Furthermore, statistics reveal that most women who practice oral contraception can be characterized as being white, college-educated, and non-Catholic. At the present time, the most prescribed oral contraceptives are Ovral, Ovulen-21, and Ortho-Novum.

Oral contraceptive drugs have gone through an interesting pattern of acceptance. When it first became known that a woman, by taking a single pill each day could, with near certainty, prevent pregnancy, physicians and laity alike agreed it was a monumental breakthrough. It was not long, however, until scientists discovered that continued use of "the pill" by some women resulted in physiological and pathological changes beyond the specific effect of preventing pregnancy. A kind of gloom prevaded the field for a while. As more evidence was gained, though, most physicians realized that these drugs were extremely useful, even though they did have some side effects.

While "the pill" has received wide-spread publicity in the news media, few people (especially men) have a basic knowledge of its composition, complications, and nutritional effects. Since the concept of "birth control" requires responsibility of both partners, it is important that both men and women be thoroughly familiar with "the pill."

COMPOSITION OF "THE PILL"

Oral contraceptive pills prevent pregancy by suppressing female ovulation. Two hormones, estrogen and progesterone, are primarily responsible for the menstrual or ovulation cycle. The level of these hormones in the bloodstream triggers certain reactions in the female's body and produces ovulation and menstration. Thus, a woman who regularly takes these pills can prevent the ripening of the ovum. Without the presence of a ripe ovum in the female's uterine cavity, pregnancy cannot occur.

Oral contraceptive pills that are available in the United States are primarily of two types: the combination type that contains both estrogen and progestational substances in all tablets, and the sequential type that contains estrogenic substances in tablets to be taken during the first portion of the menstrual cycle and estrogens plus progestational substances in tablets to be taken during the latter part of the mentrual cycle.

Some brands also provide a form of iron to be taken for five days at the end of the cycle (see figure 1). Also, as early as 1973, a third type of oral contraceptive has been available, the microdose progestogen-only product. It is important to note that the combination types are more effective in the prevention of conception but are, at the same time, substantially more prone to cause side reactions and serious complications. The recent trend in the United States is toward reducing the dose of both estrogenic and progestational substances.

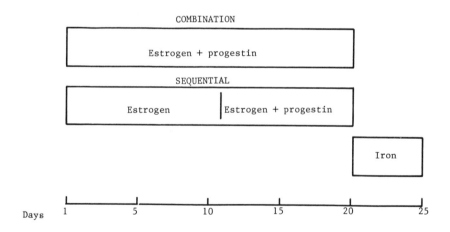

FIGURE 1. TWO TYPES OF "PILL" AND A SUPPLEMENT

Facts on Oral Contraceptives

The estrogenic substances used in oral contraceptives in the United States are either ethinyl estradiol or mestranol. On the other hand there are many different progestational compounds that differ primarily in relation to their similarity or dissimilarity to naturally occuring hormones. A variety of endocrine effects can be achieved by selecting one or another of the progestational compounds. The skillful doctor can often tailor his prescription to the individual. For example; a frail flat-chested girl who receives a compound that will, at the same time, cause breast enlargement, additional bodyweight, and effective contraception, will be pleased with the results. However, this same preparation given to a woman with a stocky build and a tendency toward hypertension might cause undesirable symptons and medical abnomalities.

COMPLICATIONS FROM "THE PILL"

The complications that result from taking oral contraceptives can be divided into two groups, those that are merely annoying and those that are serious or potentially fatal. Conditions such as nausea, vomiting, emotional changes, facial pigmentation, and slight loss of hair will occur with similar frequency in pregnant women and women taking "the pill." On the other hand, headaches are not a common accompliment of normal pregnancy, whereas they do occur more often in women taking oral contraceptives. There is some evidence to suggest that those who have migraine or similar vascular headaches may be unable to use this form of contraception.

Oral contraceptives had been used for nearly eight years before medical science presented conclusive evidence that serious and even fatal complications could result from taking "the pill." Complications are of three major types: hypertension, thromboembolic phenomena (the obstruction of a blood vessel), and diabetes mellitus.

Undoubtedly, the reason these complications were not recognized sooner is that they are relatively uncommon. In women between the ages of twenty and thirty-four, the excessive death rate from thromboembolic phenomena is in the range of 1.5 to 2.2 per 100 thousand persons per year. In women between the ages of thirty-five and forty-four years, the excessive death rate is more than doubled to 3.9 to 4.5 per 100 thousand. Even so, the morbidity and mortality rate accompanying the use of oral contraceptives remains less than 10% of that occuring in pregnancy.

TABLE 1. COMPLICATIONS FROM PREGNANCY AND USE OF ORAL CONTRACEPTIVES

CONDITION	PREGNANCY	"THE PILL"
	Minor Complications	
Nausea, vomiting	common, early	occasional
Emotional changes	occasional	occasional
Facial pigmentation	common	common
Bitemporal alopecia	slight	common
Headaches	seldom	occasional
	Serious complications	
Hypertension	seldom	seldom
Thromboembolic phenomena	rare	rare
Diabetes mellitus	seldom	seldom

NUTRITIONAL EFFECTS OF "THE PILL"

A comparison between the metabolic and nutritional effects of oral contraception and normal pregnancy is revealing (see Table 2). The weight gain during pregnancy, exclusive of the fetus, membranes, and amniotic fluid approximates ten pounds, whereas most women gain about six pounds when they begin taking oral contraceptives. There is also some fluid retention and breast enlargement in both conditions. There is also some impairment of carbohydrate metabolism.

In normal pregnancy, the nitrogen balance is positive because the fetus is storing nitrogen, but the mother herself is in negative nitrogen balance unless she pays close attention to her diet. The oral contraceptive, depending on the type selected may have slight or substantial beneficial effect in terms of nitrogen balance.

Lipid metabolism is altered during both pregnancy and with "the pill." Normal pregnancy, especially during the third trisemester, results in substantial increases of both triglyceride and cholesterol concentrations. Women taking "the pill" also have a substantial rise in triglyceride level, but there is less effect on blood cholesterol in most women.

Mineral metabolism is, however, quite different. Normal pregnancy places a severe strain on calcium metabolism and may result in irreparable damage to the teeth of a pregnant woman. Likewise, the

187

TABLE 2. COMPARISON BETWEEN NORMAL PREGNANCY AND ORAL CONTRACEPTIVES

CONDITION	NORMAL PREGNANCY	"THE PILL"
Weight gain		
Maternal	10 pounds	6 pounds
Breast enlargement	+ +	+
Fluid retention	+	+,–
Protein metabolism	+ balance	+,- balance
Carbohydrate metabolism	normal or decreased	normal or decreased
Lipid metabolism	triglycerides increased cholesterol increased	triglycerides increased, cholesterol normal or increased
Mineral metabolism	calcium decreased iron decreased	calcium stable iron increased

availability of iron is frequently less than the demands of pregnancy, resulting in a negative balance. Oral contraceptives seem to have little effect on calcium metabolism, but they do have a beneficial effect on iron metabolism. It is important to recall that some oral contraceptives include five tablets that contain an iron preparation to be taken during those days when no active hormonal substance is taken.

Other nutrients also show alteration as a result of taking oral contraceptives. Many doctors find that an essential amino acid, tryptophan, is remarkably altered. This abnormality can be largely eliminated by taking the B-vitamin, pyridoxine. Also, many oral contraceptive users are likely to become deficient in vitamin C and folic acid. To combat these deficiencies, several pharmaceutical companies have recently marketed a special vitamin and mineral preparation for oral contraceptive users. Therefore, a well-balanced diet is especially important for women taking oral contraceptives.

CONCLUSION

Medical authorities agree that outside of surgical sterilization, "the pill" is the most reliable method of contraception. Properly used it can offer 100% protection against pregnancy. However, there are certain side effects and complications from taking "the pill." The decision on whether to take "the pill," then, is one of balancing risks. Couples who decide to use this method should do so under experienced medical supervision. Remember, successful contraception requires the rational behavior and responsibility of both parties. So, read and study all you can on contraception. You can make the wisest decision if you know all the facts. And, this decision is too important to be based on rumor and hearsay.

Eat Your Way to Energy

21

EAT YOUR WAY TO ENERGY

How would you like to increase your energy as much as 300%?

Well, this is certainly possible if you follow the recommendations of this article.

Long-distance runners and cross-country skiers have used these recommendations for years with great success. But, few athletes outside of these two areas have known about them, much less used them.

What is this little-known secret? It's a special dietary routine that centers around a carbohydrate-rich diet.

The entire diet is based upon your body's ability to store and utilize GLYCOGEN. Glycogen is formed from sugar and other carbohydrate foods and is stored in the liver as well as the muscles where it is used to provide energy for muscular contraction. Thus, in long, gruelling competition, your capacity to utilize glycogen can be the difference between your winning and losing. All else being equal, increasing your glycogen utilization capacity will provide you with a substantial edge over your opponent.

I know you're wondering exactly what you do to increase your glycogen utilization capacity. That is where the special diet comes in. Before I list the specifics of this diet, I think you should know about the original research that resulted in the discovery of this diet.

In 1968 a team of Swedish scientists, headed by Dr. Jonas Bergstrom, investigated the role of glycogen stores in the body, and its function in prolonged exercise. Those taking part in the experiment were required to ride a bicycle ergometer to exhaustion, while muscle biopsies were taken from the thigh at ten-minute intervals. Chemical analysis revealed that glycogen content of the thigh muscles decreased steadily throughout the exercise. At the zero glycogen point, the subject suddenly became unable to continue.

In trying to increase glycogen reserves, the scientists fed the subjects various diets: high protein, high fat, high carbohydrate, and normal mixed. The results showed that with a high-carbohydrate diet, the maximum work capacity of a person could be increased by 300%. Thus, the high-carbohydrate diet was definitely superior as far as work capacity was concerned.

Perhaps the most important finding of the Swedish scientists concerned the storing of glycogen. When the subjects first used up their glycogen stores, and were deprived of carbohydrates for several days before being put on a high-carbohydrate diet, the muscles stored up much extra glycogen. Apparently, when a muscle is deprived of something, it overcompensates by hoarding it when it finally is replaced.

Therefore, the scientists recommended that athletes involved in sporting events exceeding thirty to sixty minutes should: deplete their glycogen stores by exercising to exhaustion the same muscles that will be used in competition (this should be done about a week prior to competition); eat almost exclusively fat and protein for the next three days; take more exercise three days prior to competition to ensure an absence of glycogen; then add large quanities of carbohydrate to the diet until competition begins. It is also important that athletes involved in prolonged competition consume weak sugar drinks between and during matches.

To simplify these recommendations, I have prepared a chart that is divided into three phases. If you are going to participate in an important event on a Saturday morning, you would begin the diet (phase II) on the preceding Sunday.

DAYS BEFORE EVENT	TRAINING	DIET
Phase 1		
8 days-Friday	Normal	Normal, mixed*
7 days-Saturday	Normal	Normal, mixed
Phase II		
6 days-Sunday	Long workout 2 1/2-3hrs.	High in protein and fat, low in carbohydrates
5 days-Monday	Rest	High in protein and fat, low in carbohydrates
4 days-Tueday	Light activity	High in protein and fat, low in carbohydrates
Phase III		
3 days-Wednesday	Hard 1 hour workout	High carbohydrate, low in protein and fat
2 days-Thursday	Rest	High carbohydrate, low in protein and fat

* United States Department of Agriculture recommends the following daily for a normal mixed diet: 2 or more servings from meat group, 2 or more servings from milk group, 4 or more servings from vegetable-fruit group, 4 or more servings from bread-cereal group.

1 day-Friday	*Rest*	*High carbohydrate, low in protein and fat*
Saturday	*Competition*	*High carbohydrate, low in protein and fat; weak sugar drinks during competition*

Here are some suggested high-fat/protein and high-carbohydrate foods:

HIGH-FAT/PROTEIN FOODS: Meat, fish, poultry, cheese, eggs, nuts, butter. It should be noted that outside of gelatin, which is almost pure protein, most protein foods contain a high percentage of fat.

HIGH-CARBOHYDRATE FOODS: Sugar, honey, candy, bread, cereals, cookies, dried fruit, potatoes (not fried), fruit and fruit juices, jams and jellies, spaghetti, and rice.

For additional dietary guidelines, refer to the table on the next page for average nutritional content of typical foods.

These nutritional guidelines apply only to the six days prior to competition. Diet and activity should be normal at other times (Phase I). Phase II lasts for three days or seventy-two hours and is immediately followed by Phase III which also lasts for three days. Best results from the program occur if the dietary recommendations are strickly practiced. "Strict" means that 90% of the diet in Phase II should be fat/protein, and 90% of the diet in Phase III should be carbohydrate. I also recommend that this diet be practiced no more than once every six weeks. Complications could result if it is practiced more frequently. Only a very important competition or tournament merits such preparation.

During normal competition and training, your glycogen utilization capacity can still be increased greatly if you frequently eat carbohydrate-rich foods. The normal diet of a competitive athlete should be composed of approximately 60% carbohydrate, 27% fat, and 13% protein. Carbohydrates are the body's preferred sources of energy, therefore the majority of an athlete's diet should be carbohydrates.

CAUTION: Athletes should avoid trying the special carbohydrate-rich diet in preparation for a major tournament without first having experimented with it prior to a minor tournament. While there have been no reported difficulties, it is possible that the diet might be unacceptable to some individuals and could cause nausea or diarrhea. Anyone comtemplating this program should get approval of their doctor.

FOOD TABLE
AVERAGE NUTRITIONAL CONTENT OF TYPICAL FOODS

The average fat content

1. Oils, shortenings	100%
2. Butter, margarine	80%
3. Most nuts	60%
4. Peanut butter, bacon, donuts	50%
5. Cheese, beef roasts	33%
6. Lunch meat, franks	27%
7. Lean pork, ice cream, cakes, pies	13%
8. Most fish, lean lamb	7%
9. Milk, shellfish, plain rolls	3%
10. Most breads	1%

The average protein content

1. Most fish, meats, cheese	25%
2. Most nuts	16%
3. Eggs	13%
4. Breads	9%
5. Legumes	7%
6. Most cake	5%
7. Milk	4%
8. Most deep green vegetables, corn, rice	3%
9. Most fruit	1%

The average carbohydrate content

1. Sugar, honey	99%
2. Most dry cereals	80%
3. Cookies, crackers	73%
4. Dried fruits, jams	70%
5. Bread	50%
6. Grains, noodles, potatoes	25%
7. Legumes, beans, peas	18%
8. Fresh fruits	12%
9. Leafy vegetables	4%

SHOWN AS A PERCENTAGE OF TOTAL WEIGHT

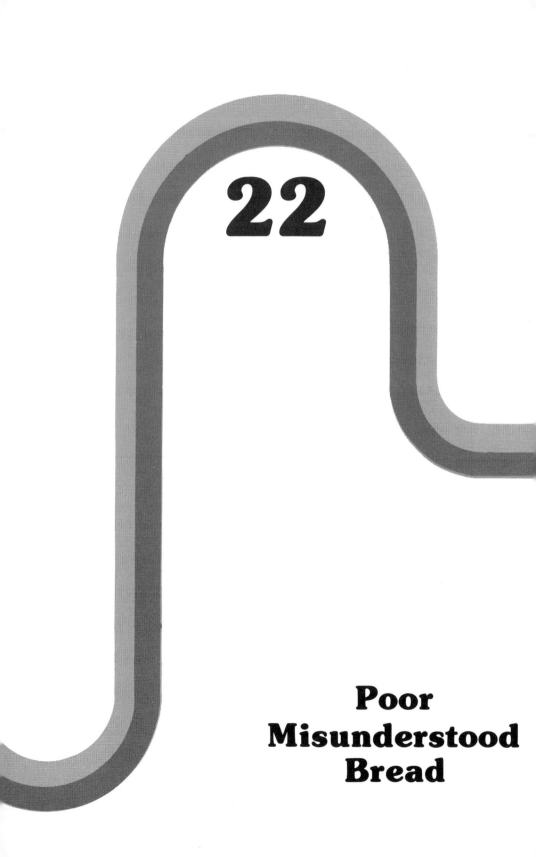

22

**Poor
Misunderstood
Bread**

POOR MISUNDERSTOOD BREAD

*When you bake all the myths in the fire of scientific
investigation, the truths rise to the surface. Finally,
here's the truth about bread.*

Bread, historically, was the veritable symbol of life— if not the
staff itself. St. Augustine, the great Christian leader of the early
church carried the concept a step further. He thought of bread in Holy
Communion as the "medicine of immortality." Today many young
adults connect the word bread with money (dough). Teenagers, on
the other hand, think of " Bread" as being the name of a popular
rock and roll group.

These many meanings of the word bread show the importance
it holds for everyone. From a health standpoint, though, its real
importance lies in its being the cornerstone of the "Basic Four Food
Groups."

Although more people eat bread today than any other foodstuff,
many misconceptions surround its nutritional value. This is epecially
true in the United States. Food faddists are constantly using such
alarming claims as "the whiter the bread, the sooner you're dead."
Nothing could be further from the truth!

It is important for us to take a look at the truth and to answer
some of the most frequently asked questions about bread. The answers to these questions will help you eliminate many misconceptions
about bread and its nutritional value.

First, how is bread made? Most of the world's bread is made
from such grains as rice, wheat, rye, barley, oats, and corn. In the
United States, though, the preference has always been for bread made
from wheat.

Originally grain was converted to flour by grinding it between
stones. This produced a flour that was coarse and grayish in appearance and made bread that was not attractive. About 1870, stone-
grinding was replaced by roller mills in which steel rollers replaced
stones. This change made possible finer milling in greater quantities
than could be done with stones.

Basic   principles of bread-making have changed little over the
years. What is done today is much the same as was done in ancient
Egypt. First, flour is moistened with water to make dough. Yeast is
then added prior to baking. If left at a warm temperature, the yeast
ferments and causes the bread to rise. Then the bread is kneaded
and put in an oven to bake where it rises once again.

Poor Misunderstood Bread

When you go into a supermarket, you see the terms "whole grain," "restored," "enriched," and "fortified" on the bread labels. Just what do these terms mean?

The term "whole grain" which can apply to wheat, rice, rye, or oats means that the entire grain has been used in the product. "Restored" and "enriched" are interchangeable terms that mean certain nutrients lost in the processing procedure (iron and three B vitamins–riboflavin, thiamin, and niacin) have been replaced to the levels found in whole grain.

When nutrients other than these are added, or the amounts added higher than the maximum levels established by the Federal government, the term "fortified" is used.

If you do alot of home baking, be sure to use enriched or whole-grain flour whenever possible. If you use convenience products, buy biscuit mixes, cake mixes, and refrigerated products that are made with enriched or whole-grain flour. Do the same with packaged rolls, saltines, and cookies.

You may wonder: why is bread enriched in the first place? In the 1920's and 1930's numerous cases of beriberi, pellagra, and riboflavin deficiency were seen in many clinics in the United States. The number of Americans suffering from B-complex deficiency was estimated to be one-third of the total population. There were over 200,000 cases of pellegra in the Southern USA, with beriberi and riboflavin deficiencies widespread. In 1928 there were 7,000 deaths in the United States from pellegra alone.

Reliable surveys of the nutritional condition of people revealed that the average American diet of the 1930's contained only one-third the amount of thiamin as when stone-ground flour was the only flour available.

As a result of these deficiencies, nutritionists started to try to convert the public to whole wheat flour from white flour. Much to the dismay of these determined nutritionists, the public continued to demand nice, attractive white bread and flour.The public seemed to be oblivious to nutrition.

Members of the medical and nutritional groups began discussing enrichment of bread and cereal products as early as 1936. However, it was not until the Nutrition Conference for Defense, in Washington, in 1941, that the national program for the enrichment of bread and flour was officially inaugurated. The enrichment of white bread was adopted as the easiest, simplest, least expensive way of restoring certain nutrients to the diets of the greatest number of people. Of the Basic Four Food Groups (meat; milk; bread and cereal; and fruit and vegatable), bread represented the most widely used of all foodstuffs. This was particularly true for those on limited food budgets.

How successful has this enrichment program been in eliminating certain nutritional diseases? In 1943 the death rate for pellegra was one per 100,000 population. Seven years later the death rate had dropped to 0.2 per 100,000. That year there were only 260 reported cases of pellegra. In 1960, data at the Hillman General Hospital in Birmingham, Alabama, revealed that not a single pellegrin was found in this area where pellegra was once rampant.

Similar findings were also recorded in a large general hospital in Chicago where beriberi was always a problem. A three-year search failed to reveal a single case of beriberi. In fact, twenty-five years after bread enrichment started in the United States, the serious deficiency diseases decreased to a point that it became difficult to find any cases at all.

However, by the latter part of the 1960's, the eating habits of this nation had changed considerably. As people became more affluent and transit, dietary habits were modified. The swing from the bread-cereal group which had been constant since 1910 increased. This caused flour consumption to drop from 200 pounds per person in 1910 to 100 pounds per person per year in the sixties. Americans gradually increased their intake of meat and sugar and decreased their consumption of bread and cereal.

The result of the reduced intake of bread and cereal was seen in the recent U.S.D.A. Ten State Nutritional Study. This study revealed a recurrence of vitamin deficiency diseases and iron deficiency anemia.

Naturally, this opened the door to the food fad promoters. Unfortunately these faddists are adept at mixing just enough established facts with fallacies to deceive unsuspecting persons.

Food faddists constantly claim the superiority of whole wheat bread over enriched white bread. While whole wheat bread is indeed nutritious, there is little nutritional difference between it and white bread that has been enriched. The obvious answer to the elimination of certain nutritional diseases is not the consumption of whole wheat bread rather than enriched white bread---but the eating of more enriched bread and cereal products.

What are the major nutritional elements of enriched bread? The major elements are niacin, riboflavin, thiamin, iron, protein, carbohydrate, and calcium. A brief description of these nutrients follows:

Niacin--helps the body utilize energy from carbohydrates and contributes to alertness.

Riboflavin—aids in growth, essential for healthy skin and eyes.

Thiamin---helps in the utilization of carbohydrates and is required to keep nerves healthy.

Iron—essential for good red blood; helps prevent anemia.

Protein—vital for good growth, strong muscles.

Carbohydrate--an ideal source of energy.

Calcium--important for strong bones, sound teeth.

Bread also contributes to our health by providing roughage in the diet. Roughage is important for intestinal functions and facilitates regular bowel movements. Also, bread is just about zero in cholesterol. With rising food prices, bread is a real bargain. Gram for gram, you will find bread costs considerably less than hamburger, cheese, potatoes, tuna, chicken, eggs, or milk.

You may wonder how bread can be enriched when milling takes out many nutrients and only four of them are replaced. It is true that levels of nutrients are decreased in milling wheat into flour. Minute amounts of sodium, magnesium, and manganese, and other trace elements are lost in milling. There are numerous food sources for these lost nutrients. Enrichment was never intended to return all the nutritional elements removed in the milling process. Enrichment was designed to correct certain nutritional deficiencies. It does that by returning the three B-vitamins and iron.

Another question frequently asked is: aren't the enrichment ingredients "chemical" and "synthetic?" Yes, but nothing is wrong with their being "chemical" and "synthetic." Unfortunately, food faddists have promoted only "natural" and "organic" vitamins and minerals as being acceptable.

This claim is utterly ridiculous! A vitamin has a certain chemical structure regardless of whether it is synthetic or natural. What most people fail to realize is that the human body is composed of chemicals--many different chemicals working together.

Why is it true that Americans prefer white bread five to one? There has always been a certain snobbery about the color of bread. For centuries the eating of white bread was considered a mark of social position in much the same way as living in a certain section of town or the possession of a Cadillac is today. The Romans were probably responsible for this. The senators and senior officers in their army took pride in providing their guests with white bread made from wheaten flour. Dark bread made from millet, barley, and other coarse grains was generally regarded as food for the working classes.

It was not long until merry ol' England followed suit. During the fourteenth century, even the peasant classes began to develop a taste for wheaten flour and a growing demand followed for better, which meant whiter, bread. Naturally, the English brought their habits and eating customs to the new world. As a result, the Americans still prefer soft, white bread in their homes.

What about the claim that whole wheat bread is superior to enriched white bread in nutritional quality? The truth is that there is basically no significant difference between the nutritional quality of whole wheat bread and enriched white bread. In fact, Dr. Fredrick Stare of the Department of Nutrition at Harvard University, stated the opinion of most nutritionists when he said: "I don't know if there is any evidence to support the idea that whole wheat products are superior nutritionally to humans compared with enriched flours."

Enriched bread with thiamin, niacin, riboflavin, iron and milk solids provides the same values as whole wheat bread does. It also gives twice as much riboflavin and a great deal more calcium because of the addition of milk solids. Therefore, where bread is concerned, you can eat what appeals to you--white, dark, French, Italian--just as long as the label states: whole grained or enriched.

Some people refuse to eat bread because they believe it is a calorie filled, fattening food. Actually, bread contains only a small number of calories. An average slice of enriched white bread contains about sixty calories. In a reducing diet, the aim is to cut down on calories while maintaining the intake of the necessary nutrients. For this reason, bread should be a basic part of every reducing diet.

The real reason most people relate bread to a fattening food is not the bread itself, but what they put on top of it. A pad of butter, for example increases the caloric value of that bread by 100 calories. Add a slice of cheese to that bread, and the calorie count goes up by an additional 115.

That cheese sandwich packs a hefty 275 calories, but the caloric contribution of the bread remains at sixty calories. It is obvious that bread itself is not fattening. Bread is simply an innocent vehicle for the high-calorie foods that people heap on top of it.

How much bread does one need a day? The Food and Nutrition Board recommends at least four servings a day from the bread-cereal group. One serving equals one slice of bread or any one of the following: 1/2 cup rice or pasta, five 2-inch saltines, one muffin, biscuit, or small roll, two pancakes, four melba toast pieces, 3/4 cup unsweetened puffed or flaked dry cereal, two graham crackers, or one cup of popcorn.

Dr. Mark Hegsted, chairman of the Food and Nutrition Board, plainly states that the American public would be better off if it would eat more bread. Certainly this would be advantageous to the average American who is suffering or will suffer from heart disease, since bread contains little fat and no cholesterol.

A big question is: how important is bread in an athlete's diet? Dr. Olaf Mickelson, professor of nutrition at Michigan State University, conducted a study that helps answer this question. He fed university athletes a predominantly enriched bread diet (eight slices per meal, three times a day, for ninety days). He found that the athletes enjoyed improved health, as measured in clinical tests, and were able to carry on an intensive program of physical activity. You see, bread does play an essential role in the diet of an athlete.

In addition, bread should be especially important to an athlete who participates in long, endurance-type activities like distance running, distance swimming, basketball, or soccer. The starch in bread is an ideal source of energy since it is slowly broken down into glucose. This prevents rapid increase in blood sugar and thus insures a more uniform production of insulin by the pancreas. In short, bread is a great boon to the energy process.

CONCLUSION

The loaf of enriched bread you buy today represents over fifty years of research. It is made from flour that satisfies the popular demand for whiteness and fine milling to improve texture. Yet, today's bread carries a full quota of the most important nutrients; (1) proteins from wheat and milk; (2) energy from starch; (3) thiamin and riboflavin; (4) niacin, the anti-pellegra vitamin; (5) calcium from milk; and (6) iron to help prevent nutritional anemia.

Yes, you will have to admit while bread can be money, music, and immortaility---- most of all it is KING OF THE BASIC FOUR!

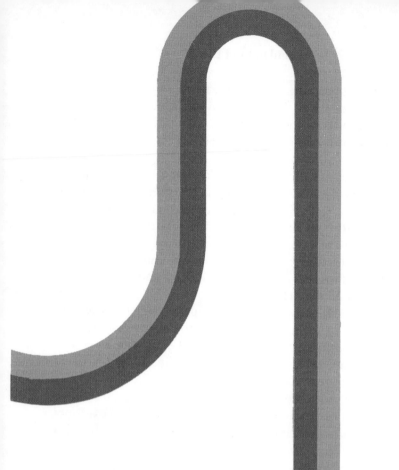

The ABC's
of Fresh Fruits
and Vegetables

23

THE ABC'S OF FRESH FRUITS AND VEGETABLES

Fruits are eaten and enjoyed by people in every country in the world.Their varied colors, ranging from red and yellow to blue and purple, are never ending sources of delight. Their numerous flavors range from the sweetness of a banana and strawberry to the tartness of the lemon and cranberry. Fruits are prized throughout the world for their health-giving properties and for the variety they add to our diet.

People often ask what is the difference between fruits and vegetables. Fruits generally are eaten raw just as they come from the plant, while vegetables are more often cooked. Crops listed as fruits are usually grown on trees, shrubs, and vines that live and produce for many years. On the other hand, vegetable crops usually live and produce a single season.

KINDS OF FRUITS

Fruits can be grouped in three classes. There are those grown in tropical, subtropical, and temperate climates. In frigid climates, a few stunted temperate-climate fruits can be grown.

Tropical Fruits. The most important tropical fruits bought and sold are bananas and pineapples. Bananas are shipped to all parts of the world as fresh fruit. Pineapples are, for the most part, sold as canned fruit or juice. Hundreds of other kinds of tropical fruits are grown and eaten by those who live in tropical countries, but few of these are marketed in other countries.

Subtropical Fruits. The most important of the subtropical fruits are the citrus ones. Included in this group are oranges, lemons, limes, tangerines, and grapefruits. Other fruits that fall into this class are figs, dates, and olives. Avocados may also be included, although they are less resistant to cold than the others.

Temperate-Zone Fruits. There are a tremendous number of fruits in this group. The most important in terms of world production are grapes and apples. Others of major importance are pears, plums, apricots, cherries, and berries such as strawberries, gooseberries, cranberries, blackberries, raspberries, and currants.

FOOD VALUE OF FRUITS

Fruits are an essential part of the human diet. Yellow and orange fruit---peaches, apricots, oranges---contribute vitamin A, which promotes normal vision, especially in dim light, and helps keep the skin and linings of the nose and mouth and inner organs in good condition. Most fruits are fair sources of B-complex vitamins, which help with steady nerves, normal appetite, and good digestion, and healthy skin.

Most of all, fruit is important as a source of vitamin C. Vitamin C helps cement body cells, keeps tissue in good condition, and helps the healing of wounds. A four-ounce glass of orange or grapefruit juice goes a long way toward meeting your daily need for vitamin C.

Although most varieties are not rich sources or iron, which helps build red blood, blackberries, apricots, peaches, prunes, figs, raisins, and dates, used in liberal amounts, are fair sources.

Fruits also contain cellulose. Because people cannot digest it, it adds bulk to the intestines, and this stimulates regular bowel movements.

WHEN TO BUY FRUIT?

Try to make the most of your fruit buying by remembering that fresh fruits are best in quality and lowest in price during the peak of their season.

SELECTING AND STORING FRUIT

Apples. They should be firm, have good color with no blemishes or soft spots. Apples can be stored in a cool, dark airy place for several weeks, but they will need occasional sorting to remove spoiled fruit. They will keep two weeks in the refrigerator in plastic bags or the hydrator.

Apricots. They should be plump, yellow-orange, and not too firm, greenish, or mushy. They will keep in the refrigerator for three to five days in a covered container or plastic bag.

Avocados. Avocados range from purple-black with a rough textured skin to green with a smooth textured skin. Be sure to look for bright, fresh-looking fruit, heavy for its size. Avoid wilted or bruised fruit with dark sunken spots or cracked surfaces. Avocados usually need three to five days ripening at room temperature, then keep in the warmest part of the refrigerator. When ripe, a toothpick passes easily through the stem end.

Bananas. They are harvested green and found in varying degrees of ripeness in your store. Your choice depends upon how you will use them. Store in the refrigerator after ripening.

Berries and Cherries. Store berries in the refrigerator without washing. When you are ready to eat them, run cold water gently over them, but do not soak.

Blueberries. Select plump, dry, dark blueberries. They should be free of stems and leaves and uniform in size.

Cherries. Sweet cherries are bright to deep red. Choose them with a fresh, ripe color. Sweet cherries are firm; sour cherries are medium firm. If they are small, hard, or have a poor color, they are less juicy. Softness, dullness, or leeking juices indicates they are overripe. Cuts are marks indicate decay.

Cranberries. They should be shiny, firm, and bright in color. They will store in the refrigerator for one to four weeks and are easily frozen in an unopened bag.

Raspberries. They should be solid, plump, and fresh. They are overripe if mushy.

Strawberries. These should be uniform in color and shape. Their caps and stems should still be in place.

Grapefruit. Small spots on the skin do not affect the quality. The fruit should be firm and heavy for its size. It may be kept a day or two at room temperature or stored in the refrigerator for several weeks.

Grapes. They should be well-formed, bright in color, and firmly attached to the stem. Darker varieties should be free of green tinge; white grapes should be amber in color. Grapes are firmly soft to the touch when they are ripe and will not ripen after picking.

Lemons and Limes. Lemons are yellow and have either a thick or thin skin. Limes have a thin green skin. Both should be firm and fresh looking and feel heavy for their size. They need not be refrigerated.

Melons. When they are ripe, they will keep for a week in the refrigerator.

Canteloupes. They are oval, grayish and covered with a thick golden netting. They have a delicate aroma when ripe.

Crenshaws. This fruit has a more pointed stem end. It is smooth, with a green-gold rind. Blossom end is soft and rind dark when ripe.

Honeydews. Honeydews are creamy white to creamy yellow with a large, velvety rind and faint fragrance when ripe.

Watermelons. They are symmetrically shaped with a dull surface and underside turning from white to a pale green to light yel-

The ABC's of Fresh Fruit and Vegetables;

Seasonal Buying Calendar for Fruits

January	February	March
Apples	Apples	Apples
Grapefruit	Grapefruit	Grapefruit
Oranges	Oranges	Oranges
Tangelos	Rhubarb	Pineapples
Tangerines	Strawberries	Rhubarb
		Strawberries

April	May	June
Apples	Grapes	Apricots
Pineapples	Rhubarb	Blueberries
Rhubarb	Strawberries	Cantaloupes
		Cherries
		Grapes
		Lemons
		Limes
		Nectarines
		Peaches
		Plums, Prunes
		Strawberries
		Watermelons

July	August	September
Apricots	Blueberries	Apples
Blueberries	Cantaloupes	Grapes
Cantaloupes	Grapes	Honeydews
Cherries	Honeydews	Nectarines
Grapes	Limes	Peaches
Lemons	Nectarines	Pears
Limes	Peaches	Prunes
Nectarines	Pears	
Peaches	Plums, Prunes	
Plums, Prunes	Watermelons	
Watermelons		

October	November	December
Apples	Apples	Apples
Cranberries	Cranberries	Cranberries
Grapes	Grapes	Grapefruit
Pears	Tangelos	Oranges
		Tangelos
		Tangerines

This chart will give you
a good idea of the optimum time to buy
fresh fruits. Remember: the taste is best and the cost
is less when you buy fruits at the peak of their season.

low when ripe.

Oranges. Their skin color is not an indication of quality. They should be firm, heavy for size, without soft or discolored spots, cuts, or skin punctures. Can be kept cold or at room temperature.

Peaches. Peaches are fairly round with velvety skin. They should be plump, fairly firm and creamy to yellowish in color with a red blush. Keep them unwashed in the refrigerator.

Nectarines. This fruit should be bright looking, plump, and yellow-orange between the red area. Pick the fruit firm to moderately hard and allow to ripen two to three days at room temperature. Avoid hard, dull, or slightly shriveled fruit or that with cracks or bruises. Russeting of skin does not affect the eating quality.

Pears. Pick them hard and allow to ripen at room temperature. They should be plump, fairly firm, and free from bruises. Eat while firm, as they ripen from inside out. Keep cold and humid.

Pineapples. Buy when heavy for size and as large as possible. You get a greater portion of edible flesh. Check bottom for signs of decay. Crown leaves should be fresh and dark green. Avoid fruit with soft spots or sunken pips. These will keep two or three days in the refrigerator.

Plums. Their color is not an indication of quality. They should be smooth, fairly firm to slightly soft with no cracks. Ripen, then store covered in the refrigerator.

Rhubarb. Stalks should be firm, crisp with a bright color. Never eat the leaves. Refrigerate immediately and use within two days since it is highly perishable.

Tangerines. They should be deep orange to almost red color with a bright luster. Should be heavy for the size with a puffy appearance. Keep cold and use and soon as possible.

FREEZING FRESH FRUITS

Fruit to be frozen should be firm and ripe. Most fruits freeze with a texture similar to that of fresh fruit but generally softer.

Carefully washed fruits may be frozen in syrup, sugar, or unsweetened. Most fruits are best using either the syrup or sugar method.

In the sugar pack, simply mix sugar and fruit until it is dissolved. A small piece of water-resistant paper should be crumpled on top to hold the fruit under the juice in packing.

The ABC's of Fresh Fruits and Vegetables

GUIDELINES FOR FREEZING FRESH FRUITS

Fruit	Preparation	Pack
Avocadoes	Wash, peel, pit and mash soft ripe fruit.	Add ascorbic acid or ¼ cup lime juice for each pint of mashed avocado.
Banana	Peel, mash or puree.	Add ascorbic acid powder or ¼ cup lemon juice for each pint mashed banana.
Berries and Strawberries	Sort, wash and drain, cap. Freeze small berries whole. Slice or crush large berries if desired.	Syrup pack in 40 to 50 per cent syrup. Sugar pack -- 1 cup sugar to 5 cups fruit. Unsweetened pack -- pack fruit and omit sugar.
Carambola	Wash, trim dark spiny edges, slice cross ways.	Syrup pack in 40 to 50 per cent syrup. Sugar pack 1 cup sugar to 5 cups fruit. Unsweetened pack -- pack fruit, omit sugar.
Carissa	Wash, peel if desired, cut in half lengthwise or leave whole.	Syrup pack in 40 to 50 per cent syrup.
Cherries Barbados	Wash, remove stems, blender chop, press through cheesecloth.	Add 1 cup sugar and 1 tablespoon liquid pectin to each 2 cups pureed fruit.
Cherries Surinam	Wash, remove stem and seeds.	Syrup pack in 40 to 50 per cent syrup. Sugar pack -- 1 cup sugar to 5 cups fruit. Unsweetened pack -- pack fruit, omit sugar.
Grapefruit or Orange	Wash, peel, section fruit removing all membrane and seeds.	Syrup pack in 40 per cent syrup. Add ascorbic acid if desired. Unsweetened pack -- pack fruit, omit sugar.
Coconut	Clean, shred, grind or blender chop.	Cover with coconut milk. Add two tablespoon sugar for each cup of coconut.
Figs	Wash, sort, remove stems, drain.	Syrup pack in 30 per cent syrup.
Loquats	Wash, remove stem and blossom end, remove seeds.	Syrup pack in 30 per cent syrup.
Lychee	Wash, remove shells and seeds.	Syrup pack in 40 to 50 per cent syrup or dry pack whole in shell.
Guava	Wash, peel thinly, cut in halves.	Syrup pack in 50 to 60 per cent syrup.
Grapes	Wash, stem and seed, freeze in halves.	Syrup pack halves in 40 per cent syrup or pack without sugar.
	Puree or juice -- wash, stem and crush grapes. Heat to boiling. Drain off free juice and freeze. Cool crushed grapes and press through sieve.	Pack juice with or without sugar. Add ½-cup sugar to each quart of puree.
Mango	Wash, peel, slice. Freeze in slices or blender chop and freeze puree.	Arrange on flat pan and freeze. Remove when frozen and store in sealed containers. Syrup pack in 30 per cent syrup. Freeze puree with or without sugar.
Peaches	Sort, wash, pit and peel. Cut in halves, slices or puree in blender.	Syrup pack in 40 per cent syrup. Add ascorbic acid or two tablespoons lemon juice for each pint of peaches.
Pears	Wash, peel, core and slice in pieces. Place slices in boiling water 1 to 3 minutes. Drain and cool.	Syrup pack in 40 per cent syrup. Add ascorbic acid or two tablespoons lemon juice for each pint of pears (optional).
Persimmons	Wash, peel, cut into sections; blender chop or press through sieve.	Add ascorbic acid or two tablespoons lemon juice for each pint. Needs no sugar.

The ABC's of Fresh Fruits and Vegetables

TYPE OF SYRUP	CUPS SUGAR	CUPS WATER	CUPS YIELD
30% syrup	2	4	5
40% syrup	3	4	5 1/2
50% syrup	4 3/4	4	6 1/2
60% syrup	7	4	7 3/4

To prevent discoloration of lighter fruits, the addition of ascorbic acid (vitamin C) or citric acid in cyrstalline or powder form is suggested. Follow the directions on the package.

Fruits properly packaged and kept under zero degrees storage are safe to use up to eight to twelve months; citrus fruits should be eaten in four to six months.

See "Guidelines for Freezing Fresh Fruits" on page 208.

FRESH VEGETABLES

Fresh vegetables are more important in supplying our food needs than they have ever been before. There are two reasons for this: one, modern transportation allows us to have a wide variety of vegetables all year long; two, we understand the kinds of foods the body needs much better than our grandfathers did.

The production of vegetables is an important part of American agriculture. Market gardeners and truck farmers grow vegetables and ship them by refrigerator trucks to all parts of the country. In addition, vegetables are grown indoors in greenhouses during the winter in the northern part of the United States so that there is a constant supply.

Vegetables are important to us because of the vitamins and minerals they contain. They are especially rich in vitamin A, thiamen, niacin, and vitamin C. They are also important sources of vital minerals, including calcium, phosphorus, and iron. Vegetables give bulk to the diet, and this helps our digestive process. Nutritionists recommend that in addition to one serving of potatoes, we eat one green leafy vegetable and one yellow vegetable a day.

SEASONAL BUYING

Vegetables are highest in quality and lowest in price in peak season. Therefore, let us examine the vegetables which are plentiful during different months. Cabbage, carrots, onions, and potatoes, which are available all year, are not included.

SELECTING AND STORING VEGETABLES

Artichokes. Since you buy them by the unit, get as large of one as you can. Leaves should be compact, tightly closed, plump, and green. Loose-spreading or discolored leaves are a sign of poor quality and over-maturity. They will keep four days in the refrigerator in a covered container or plastic bag.

Asparagus. Look for straight, green, brittle stalks that break easily. Tips that have begun to spread show over-maturity. Wilted, thin or crooked stalks may be tough or stingy. Asparagus keeps, unwashed for four days in the refrigerator in a covered container.

Beans (snap). Look for crisp beans, free from scars and avoid dry looking pods. May be stored washed or unwashed for three to five days in a covered container in the refrigerator.

Beets. Choose deep red colored beets of uniform size with no ridges or blemishes. Do not buy any with soft spots. Tops, if any, should be fresh and green. These tops can be cooked like spinach. Beets can be kept, covered, in the refrigerator for up to two weeks.

Broccoli. Heads should be quite green or have a slight purplish color. If starting to flower or turn yellowish, they are too mature. Can be stored, covered, in the refrigerator for up to four days.

Cabbage. Leaves should be solid and well-packed and heads heavy for their size. Avoid heads that have wilted or discolored outer leaves. Raw, uncut cabbage will keep from seven to eight days in the refrigerator. Never overcook cabbage.

Carrots. Fresh carrots are firm. Large ones may have a sharp, unpleasant taste. Very tiny new carrots are tender and sweet. Buy bright orange carrots and avoid those with bumps and cracks. These will keep in the refrigerator for several weeks.

Cauliflower. It should have a firm, tight head and clean white flowerlets. If leaves have grown through the flowerlets, it does not affect the taste. Do not buy when flowerlets look grainy, or ricelike, or when leaves have yellowed or withered. It will keep in the refrigerator for several weeks.

Celery. The outer stalks should have a standard clipped length and fresh green leaves. Avoid cracked, bruised, or stringy stalks. Clean celery when you bring it home.

Corn. The husk should be bright green, tight to cob with darkbrown silk at the end. Kernels should be in even rows, and firm

The ABC's of Fresh Fruit and Vegetables

Seasonal Buying Calendar for Vegetables

January	February	March
Brussels sprouts	Belgian endive	Artichokes
Celery	Broccoli	Asparagus
Parsnips	Brussels sprouts	Belgian endive
Turnips, rutabagas	Celery	Broccoli
		Celery

April	May	June
Artichokes	Artichokes	Asparagus
Asparagus	Asparagus	Beans, snap
Belgian endive	Cauliflower	Beets
Peas, green	Corn, sweet	Corn, sweet
		Cucumbers
		Okra
		Peas, green
		Radishes
		Tomatoes

July	August	September
Beans, snap	Beats	Beets
Beets	Corn, sweet	Eggplant
Corn, sweet	Eggplant	Okra
Cucumbers	Okra	
Okra	Tomatoes	
Tomatoes		

October	November	December
Brussels sprouts	Brussels sprouts	Brussels sprouts
Cauliflower	Cauliflower	Celery
Parsnips	Celery	Endive
Pumpkins	Sweet potatoes	Sweet potatoes
Sweet potatoes	Turnips, rutabagas	
Turnips, rutabagas		

This chart will give you
a good idea of the optimum time to buy
fresh vegetables. Cabbage, carrots, onions, and
potatoes are not included because they are available all year.

enough to resist slight pressure. Store in the refrigerator without removing husks.

Cucumbers. They should be nicely shaped, firm, bright green. Yellow and puffy ones are overripe, and those with a shriveled skins are tough and bitter. Wash, dry, and store in the refrigerator up to two weeks.

Eggplant. They should be firm and smooth with a shiny, dark purple color, slightly oblong in shape. Brown, rough or spongy spots will quickly spoil the whole eggplant. Can be refrigerated up to one week.

Lettuce. When buying iceberg and romaine, look for clean crisp leaves with no ragged brown areas. Heads of iceberg should be firm. Butterhead and loose leaf lettuce should be clean, fresh, and tender with no wilting. Refrigerate immediately. Wash, clean, and remove the core, and store in a plastic bag in the refrigerator. Can be kept up to one week in the refrigerator.

Mushrooms. They should be white to creamy white with firm tops and pale beige stems. Fluted section under the top should be light in color. Brown or black color indicates old age. Store unwashed in a shallow pan and cover with a damp towel. Allow air to circulate around them and place in the refrigerator. They keep about a week.

Onions. Green onions should come in bunches with fresh, green tops. Wash carefully and peel away bruised leaves. Avoid yellow, badly damaged tops. Keep cold and humid in the refrigerator.

Dry onions have a dry, paper-thin outer skin. They should be clean, hard, and well-shaped. Moisture at the neck indicates decay. Store in a cool dry place.

Parsnips. They should be firm, smooth, and well-formed. Small or medium sized ones are best. Large ones may have wooly or pithy cores.

Peas. Pods should be uniformly green, velvety, shiny clean, and snap open easily. Flat, dark green pods indicate lack of maturity. Avoid wet, mildewed pods. Peas must be kept cool.

Peppers. Look for those that are bright red or green, have a shiny skin, and feel heavy for their size. Avoid wilted, flabby peppers with thin walls.

Potatoes. Choose firm, not wrinkled or leathery looking potatoes, free from spots or sprouting. Blackheart can be found only by cutting, but is more likely in large potatoes. Store in a cool, dark, well-ventilated place.

Radishes. They should be smooth and firm without black spots or pitting. Very large or flabby ones are likely to have pithy centers and poor flavor. Tops, if any, should be fresh and green. They may be eaten.

Spinach. It has leaves that are either flat or curly, but they should be large, crisp, and dark green. Spinach should be refrigerated in a plastic bag in the refrigerator. Avoid leaves that are wilted or blemished.

Squash. Summer squash should be fresh, tender, and fairly heavy in relation to size. It should be refrigerated. Softness in winter squash indicates immaturity and thin flesh. Store in cool dry place.

Sweet Potatoes. They should well-shaped, smooth and have uniformly colored skin. Decay may either be a soft, wet area, or a dry, shriveled, sunken, discolored area. Never store in the refrigerator.

Tomatoes. Select those that are well-formed, smooth, free from blemishes. If fully ripe, look for a red color and a slight softness. Usually better if ripened at home at room temperature until deep red. Then store in the refrigerator, but don't freeze.

Turnips and Rutabagas. Look for a smooth, fairly firm vegetable without skin puncture and obvious fibrous roots. Remove wax, if any, before cooking.

Watercress and Parsley. Look for crisp, bright green leaves. Avoid wilted or yellow bunches. Wash several times in cold water and keep cold and humid.

PREPARATION OF VEGETABLES

Preparation of vegetables usually causes some loss of nutritive value. Removal of dark outer green leaves causes a loss of vitamin A, but removal of coarse stems which are low in nutrients shortens the cooking time. Peeling before boiling increases the loss of vitamin C in potatoes but not from carrots. Cutting them into pieces of large or moderate size may result in vitamin C retention because, although it increases the soluble nutrients, it shortens cooking time.

In cooking vegetables, nutritionists recommend that a medium amount of water be used. Generally speaking, this means half to one cup of water for four servings of vegetables depending upon the vegetables being cooked. Any utensil that has a well-fitting lid and is heavy enough to prevent excessive loss of steam is suitable for retention of water soluble nutrients.

FREEZING FRESH VEGETABLES

Freezing is the simplest, cheapest, and generally speaking, the most satisfactory method of putting up that home garden bounty or vegetable stand/produce department special. All it takes is freezer space, attention to a few directions, and some fast work to capture all the fresh quality of the vegetables.

For best results, freeze only the freshest and tenderest vegetables and plan to freeze them as soon as possible after harvesting.

Most vegetables must be blanched before freezing to stop enzyme action which hastens aging and to prevent off-flavors from developing.

It is important to blanch a small amount at a time. For each pound of prepared vegetable, use one gallon of boiling water. Lower the basket containing the vegetable into the boiling water, put the lid on the kettle, and begin timing as soon as the water returns to a rolling boil.

It is equally important that the product be cooled quickly. You should plunge the basket of blanched vegetables immediately into cold water, using either running tap water or iced water. A rule of thumb is that it should take as long to to cool as it did to blanch the vegetable.

The freezer life of properly packaged vegetables is from eight to twelve months.

CONCLUSION

It is important to realize that even with the rising food prices most fruits and vegetables are excellent nutritional bargains. The malnourished American is the result of poor selection of food, not of unavailable food. You can prevent the possiblity of you or your family being malnourished by learning these ABC's of fresh fruits and vegetables.

GUIDELINES FOR FREEZING FRESH VEGETABLES

Vegetable	Preparation	Pack
Beans, bush or pole	Wash, remove ends, cut in 1- to 2-inch pieces or French cut. Blanch for 3 minutes. Chill.	Pack in containers leaving ½-inch headspace; seal and freeze.
Cabbage (suitable for cooked cabbage only)	Remove coarse outer leaves, cut into medium shreds or thin wedges, blanch for 1½ minutes. Chill.	Pack in containers leaving ½-inch headspace; Seal and freeze.
Carrots	Select tender, mild-flavored carrots. Remove tops, wash and peel. Leave small carrots whole. Cut others in ¼-inch cubes, slices or strips. Blanch whole carrots 5 minutes, slices 2 minutes. Chill.	Pack in containers leaving ½-inch headspace; seal and freeze.
Celery	Wash, trim and cut stalks into 1-inch lengths. Blanch 3 minutes in boiling water. Chill.	Pack in containers leaving ½-inch headspace; seal and freeze.
Sweet Corn	Cut corn: husk, silk, and wash. Scald 4 minutes and chill. Cut kernels at about 2/3 the depth of kernels. For cream-style cut kernels at about the center of the kernels. Scrape cobs to remove juice and heart of the kernel.	Pack in containers leaving ½-inch headspace: seal and freeze.
	On the cob: husk, silk and wash. Sort according to size, blanch 4 minutes and chill.	Wrap in air-tight moisture resistant material; seal and freeze.
Eggplant	Wash, peel and cut into 1/3 or 1/2 inch slices. Dip into solution of 1 tablespoon lemon juice to 1 quart water. Blanch 4 minutes. Chill. Dip again into lemon juice solution.	Pack in air tight containers, leaving ½-inch headspace; seal and freeze.
Greens	Select young, tender leaves. Wash well. Remove tough stems and imperfect leaves. Blanch 2 to 3 minutes. Chill.	Pack in containers leaving ½-inch headspace: seal and freeze.
Okra	Wash, remove stems, do not break seed pod. Blanch 3 to 4 minutes, chill.	Pack in containers leaving ½-inch headspace; seal and freeze.
Onions whole	Peel and wash whole onions, do not blanch.	Pack in air-tight containers, seal and freeze. Note: onions may be removed from freezer and grated in frozen state.
Mushrooms	Wash, cut off ends and stems. Slice or leave whole. Blanch large whole mushrooms 5 minutes; slices 2 to 3 minutes. Chill. Pre-cook in butter or margarine until nearly done. Air cool or set the skillet in cold water. Freeze in buttery juice.	Pack in containers leaving ½-inch headspace; seal and freeze.
Peas, green or blackeye	Shell, discard immature and tough peas. Blanch 1½ to 2 minutes, chill.	Pack raw peppers in containers leaving no headspace; seal and freeze.
Peppers, sweet	Peppers may be frozen without blanching. Wash, remove seeds, leave in halves or cut in smaller pieces.	Pack in containers leaving ½-inch headspace; seal and freeze.

215

Vegetable	Preparation	Pack
Potatoes	Wash, bake. Remove inside, mash, season with butter, milk, and salt. Return to shell. Chill. Wash, peel, cut and blanch new potatoes -- 1 inch in diameter, 6 minutes; over 1½ inches, 8-10 minutes. Chill and package. Slice in cubes. French fry. Remove before brown. Chill.	Place in air-tight wrap; seal and freeze.
Pumpkin	Wash, cut into quarters or smaller pieces and remove seeds. Cook in water until soft. Remove pumpkin rind and mash. Chill.	Pack in containers leaving ½-inch headspace; seal and freeze.
Squash summer	Wash, cut in ½-inch slices. Blanch 3 minutes. Chill.	Pack in containers leaving ½-inch headspace; seal and freeze.
Squash winter	Wash, cut into cubes and remove seeds. Cook in water until tender. Remove squash from rind and mash. Chill.	Pack in containers leaving ½-inch headspace; seal and freeze.
Sweet Potatoes	Wash, cook until tender. Peel;cut in halves, slice or mash. To prevent darkening dip slices in lemon water (½ cup lemon juice, 1 quart water). Add 2 tablespoons citrus juice to each quart of mashed sweet potatoes.	Pack in containers leaving ½-inch headspace; seal and freeze.
Tomatoes	Remove stem ends. Peel if desired. Blender chop or cut in small pieces.	Pack in containers leaving ½-inch headspace; seal and freeze.

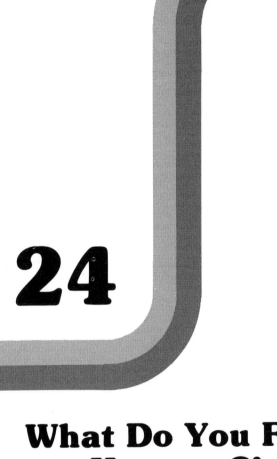

24

What Do You Feed a Hungry Girl? Nutrition Facts... That's What!

WHAT DO YOU FEED A HUNGRY GIRL?
Nutritional Facts----That's What!

Food, teenagers, nutrition, women, athletics, all of these words are important to you: the coach.

If your teenage athletes are eager eaters, you worry that they are eating the wrong things. If they are meager eaters, you worry about malnutrition. Either way, you worry that inconsistant eating habits will affect their performance on the athletic field. Unfortunately, you could be right.

Teenage girls are notoriously weight-conscious. In their efforts to stay trim, they have probably developed the poorest eating habits of all age groups. Even girls who know the rules of the eating game often chose to ignore them.

That's not all you have to worry about. Remember the "old wives' tales" about food that are constantly cropping up in the locker room or on the practice field. What of the modern-day myths that have grown up in the wake of consumer concerns? They negatively influence coaches and athletes in many ways. An example is the woman who spends her money on the latest "magic pills" that are guaranteed to give her more stamina.

This isn't a very encouraging picture, is it? How can you, as a coach, help turn the tide for your athletes? With patience. With persistance. With practical knowledge about nutrition and athletic performance.

Let's examine some of the most frequently asked questions that coaches have about food and nutrition. Based on the latest government data and information from qualified sources, the answers to these questions should provide you with substantial knowledge.

1. WHAT IS THE CHIEF FUNCTION OF FOOD? You eat food primarily to provide energy for your cells whether you are an athlete, a non-athlete, or something in between. Of course, food also has other important functions such as building and maintaining tissue and muscle mass, creating healthy blood to transport oxygen to cells, and healing wounds and broken bones. Nevertheless, the chief function of food is to supply energy.

2 .WHAT IS ENERGY AND WHERE DOES IT COME FROM? Energy is the internal power you must have for everything you do. That is right---everything----from breathing to moving, from digesting to sleeping. This even includes expressing joy or anger.

What Do You Feed A Hungry Girl?

The sun is our source of energy. In high school we learned that energy could not be created or destoyed. This is still true. We can only change its form and the place where it is available.

Only plants have the ability to grow by combining the energy from the sun with the elements from the air and soil and water. Animals get their energy originally from plants, and we get our energy from plants and from animals. From a nutritional viewpoint, food and energy are measured in calories.

3. HOW MANY CALORIES DO FEMALE ATHLETES FROM 12 TO 18 YEARS OLD NEED A DAY? The number of calories your athletes need a day depends upon their age, size, and activity. As a general rule of thumb, your athletes can get an idea of their daily caloric needs by using the following figures:

AGE	12-14 years	14-16 years	16-18 years
CALORIES per pound per day	24	21	19

For example, if Karen is fifteen and weighs 114 pounds, she needs about 2,400 calories (114 X 21= 2,400) a day to supply her energy and growth needs. Of course, these are not rigid guidelines. More or less active girls will adjust their calories per pound accordingly.

4. WHAT TYPES OF FOODS SHOULD BE EATEN DAILY BY FEMALE ATHLETES 12 TO 18 YEARS OLD? The foods they should eat daily are divided into four groups:

2 or more servings from the meat group

4 cups of dairy products

4 or more servings of fruits and vegetables

4 or more servings of breads and cereals

Plus, other foods to complete meals and provide additional energy. Some of these are butter, margarine, oils, sugar, and sweets.

Varied selections from these four basic food groups form the backbone of a balanced diet. These guidelines have received firm support from the American Medical Association for the last twenty years.

5. WHAT HABITS SHOULD I ENCOURAGE TO GET THE BEST PERFORMANCE FROM MY ATHLETES? Encourage each athlete to assume personal responsibility for a year-round schedule of regular exercise, sleep, and well-balanced meals. Insist that your athletes eat breakfast.

6. WHY IS BREAKFAST SUCH AN IMPORTANT MEAL? Breakfast is considered an important meal because it marks the end of an overnight fast. Studies made on the value of breakfast have shown that performances during the late morning and afternoon of those who skip breakfast are impaired. Breakfast, therefore, is essential for an athlete who is engaged in vigorous physical activity and who must maintain a high plane of nutrition if she is to compete at maximum capability. An adequate breakfast should supply at least 25% of your athlete's nutrient needs for the day.

7. SHOULD SPECIAL TYPES AND AMOUNTS OF FOODS BE SERVED AT A PRE-GAME MEAL? The meal before any sporting event should be acceptable to the individual athlete. Whatever an athlete feels will help her performance should be eaten.

8. DOES THE PRE-GAME MEAL SUPPLY ALL THE ENERGY FOR THE GAME? No, in fact the pre-game meal for 98% of your athletes supplies very little of the actual energy that is used in the game. The energy used ordinarily comes from food consumed from two to fourteen days prior to the contest.

The only exceptions to this rule are athletes who participate in continuous activities that last at least forty-five minutes, like long-distance running. Pre-contest meals made up of carbohydrate-rich foods can definitely add additional energy to these athletes. A carbohydrate-rich meal might include dried fruit, a jelly sandwich, cookies, and a sugar drink.

9. HOW LONG BEFORE THE GAME SHOULD THE PRE-GAME MEAL BE EATEN TO ALLOW FOR DIGESTION TO TAKE PLACE? A three to four hour period is suffcient for most athletes.

10. SHOULD LIQUID FORMULA DIETS BE SERVED AS A PRE-GAME MEAL? The liquid formula drinks are not recommended as a substitute for whole food. They can, however, be used as supplemental feeding for such events as track and field and swimming when meals are difficult to schedule. Be sure that each athlete likes the kind of supplement to be used.

11. WHAT ABOUT CARBOHYDRATE-LOADING DIETS I'VE READ ABOUT? Even though there are some risks involved in the carbohydrate-loading diet (such as nausea and diarrhea), some of your long-distance runners may want to try it. If they do, they should do so under the advice from doctors and trainers who are experienced in the technique. Remember: most athletic events are of such short duration that no benefit would be obtained from carbohydrate-loading. Only continuous activities that last at least forty-five minutes (not sports that involve stopping and starting), would be benefited.

For those of you who are unfamiliar with the concept of carbohydrate loading, this procedure involves exercising the muscles (for a runner, the lower body) one week in advance to exhaust glycogen (energy) stores. The diet is then modified to be almost exclusively fat and protein for three days to keep the glycogen content of the exercised muscles low. For the next three days, large quanities of carbohydrate-rich foods are added to the diet. As a result, the body over-compensates by storing more glycogen than would otherwise be possible.

12. WHY DOES CARBOHYDRATE-LOADING WORK? Because high-carbohydrate diets give the best energy yield per liter of oxygen compared to high-fat, high-protein, and normal-mixed diets. Also, when carbohydrate-loading is practiced properly, glycogen stores in the working muscles are increased. The importance of the high initial level of muscle glycogen is that it enables the athlete who competes in an endurance-type event to maintain her optimal pace for an extended time.

13. WHAT ARE "POWER-PACKED" AND "GO-POWER" PROTEIN PRODUCTS? WILL THEY HELP AN ATHLETE? The promotion of "power-packed" and "go-power" protein is nothing more than a sales gimmick. Although proteins can be used as energy sources if necessary, energy is almost always provided by carbohydrates and fats. These two nutrients are much preferred as energy sources since they are more easily utilized by the body. They are also cheaper than protein.

14. DO ATHLETES NEED PROTEIN PILLS? No, with a capital "N". Studies show that if an athlete gets anything out of her diet, she gets MORE than enough protein.

15. HOW MUCH PROTEIN SHOULD A FEMALE ATHLETE BE EATING A DAY? Since protein is measured in grams, you should know what a gram is. A gram is the basic unit of weight in the metric system and is equal to about 1/28 of an ounce. There are 454 grams in a pound. Food composition tables list protein in grams. For example: eight ounces of milk contain nine grams of protein, a large egg contains six grams, and a six ounce steak contains forty-eight grams. Be sure and examine food composition tables for complete listings.

Getting back to the question——nutritionists have devised a simple rule of thumb to determine adequate protein levels for female athletes. They recommend 0.8 grams of protein daily for each kilogram of body weight or .39 grams of protein for each pound of body weight. You can determine your athletes' needs by multiplying their weight by .39.

16. HOW CAN A DIET BE USED TO COMBAT HEAT STROKE? Coaches should urge their athletes to drink liberal amounts of liquids before, during, and after practice sessions, and to salt their foods. During hot weather, your athletes should be weighed before and after practice. Weight loss is probably the easiest way to measure heat acclimatization. If there is more than a 5% weight loss, watch the athlete carefully and encourage fluid replacement with a saline solution.

17. ARE SALT TABLETS OR SALINE SOLUTION BETTER FOR CONDITIONING TO HEAT? Saline solution (salted water) is more readily available to meet the need of the body. In excessive sweating, water is always lost more than salt, and fluid replacement is essential. Furthermore, salt tablets may cause irritation to the stomach lining or be passed completely undissolved.

18. HOW IS A SALINE SOLUTION MADE? A simple formula for saline solution that costs about fifteen cents a gallon is: one gallon of water, one tablespoon iodized salt, three tablespoons sugar, one package of Kool-Aid for color, ice to chill.

19. HOW MUCH AND WHEN SHOULD SALINE SOLUTION BE GIVEN? As a general rule, each athlete should be given ten to twenty ounces (one to three glasses) per hour. Once again, your athletes should be encouraged to drink before, during, and after practice. Once they become accustomed to the heat, a liberal use of water and salted food is sufficient.

20. ARE PIZZAS AND HAMBURGERS BAD FOR ATHLETES? I know some coaches are going to cringe when I say this, but there is nothing "bad" about your athletes eating pizzas and hamburgers. Properly prepared with meat or sausage, cheese, tomatoes, and enriched bread or dough, they are good sources or protein and calcium and also contribute their share of iron, vitamins A, C, and B-complex, carbohydrates, and fat to the diet.

21. WHAT ABOUT "HEALTH" FOODS? First the so-called

"health" foods are not vital for good nutrition. Nutritional scientists have been unable to find any difference between "health" foods and the foods that are at your local supermarket. All the claims and promises of "health" foods are merely clever sales gimmicks.

Also, "health" foods usually cost two to three times as much as regular foods. Have your athletes save their money.

22. WHAT DO YOU RECOMMEND FOR A WOMAN WHO NEEDS TO LOSE WEIGHT? Actually the words "lose weight" are misleading for an athlete can, and many of them do, lose weight without losing fat. Female athletes need as much muscle as they can get, but they would perform much better with a reduced percentage of body fat.

In order to reduce body fat, the body must be forced to burn its own fat as a source of energy. An athlete who consumes 500 less calories a day than her maintenance level will burn about a pound of fat a week (3,500 calories in a pound of fat) as a source of energy. This 500 calorie a day reduction should come from NO ONE food group. It should come from all the food groups. In other words, smaller servings should be eaten.

A teenage girl who loses over two pounds a week on a "crash diet" can be sure that most of the weight will be from her muscles and organs, not from her fat stores. Anything more than a two-pound weight loss a week is dangerous. Insist that your overweight girls stick to a well-balanced, lower calorie diet.

23. WHAT ABOUT GAINING WEIGHT? Once again, gaining weight is one thing, gaining muscle is totally different. I am assuming that you want your athletes to gain muscle, not fat, since fat contributes nothing to an athlete's performance.

A pound of muscle contains about 600 calories (and a lot of water), but eating an extra 600 calories will not make any difference as far as building muscle is concerned unless the athlete has stimulated muscular growth beforehand. Muscular growth is best stimulated by a program of progressive resistance exercises performed in a high-intensity fashion. For addition guidelines see the articles on strength training in Part A.

Most women, because of hormonal differences, cannot develop large muscles, at least not ones as large as men's. But, they can significantly strengthen their muscles with proper exercise.

24. WHAT ABOUT MILK? DOES IT REALLY MAKE SOME PEOPLE SICK? All athletes should have some dairy products every day. It is true, however, that some people are allergic to the lactose in milk. Recent findings show that up to 75% of black athletes have this problem.

Have athletes that cannot tolerate milk try other dairy products in which the lactose has either been removed or altered (converted to lactic acid) through fermentation. Yogurt, buttermilk, and cheese fall in this category. You might also have them try skimmed and powdered milk.

25. DOES MILK CAUSE "COTTONMOUTH"? There is no scientific evidence that milk causes "cottonmouth". "Cottonmouth" is usually a result of tension. Tension causes the salivary glands to increase the flow of saliva. As a result, the mouth becomes dry and feels fuzzy. Water, ice, and soft drinks, and chewing gum are effective in combating this condition.

26. SHOULD VITAMIN AND MINERAL PILLS BE ROUTINE— LY GIVEN TO ATHLETES? No! A balanced diet made up of the previously described four food groups will provide all the nutrients needed by athletes.

Some supplemental nutrients that are in excess of bodily requirements are merely eliminated. Therefore, they are a waste of money. Excessive intakes of certain nutrients, such as vitamin A and D, may be harmful, since they are stored in the body.

27. WILL VITAMIN E IN LARGE DOSES IMPROVE STAMINA? Vitamin E is a necessary nutrient, but taking it in large amounts will not improve an athlete's stamina. This is just another myth that surrounds the athletic world.

28. WHAT ABOUT VITAMIN C TABLETS? WILL THEY PRE- VENT COLDS? The value of vitamin C in preventing colds is still controversial. Most nutrition experts note that massive doses (up to 5000 mg. in pill form a day) can cause diarrhea, excessive urination, and kidney and bladder stones. Also, they question its value in preventing colds.

Until more conclusive evidence is available, the athlete need not consume more than the normal daily vitamin C requirement. This is easily gotten from four servings of fruits and vegetables.

29. SINCE MANY WOMEN HAVE IRON DEFICIENCIES, SHOULD WOMEN ATHLETES TAKE IRON PILLS? Many women are deficient in iron. If an athlete shows signs of unusual fatigue about mid-season, she should be sent to a doctor to have her hemoglobin checked. If the iron in her blood is low, the doctor will prescribe the appropriate iron supplement.

Since the body can only absorb about one-tenth of the iron consumed, females need 18 mg. of iron a day to extract 1 mg. to 2 mg. Good sources of iron are meats, enriched bread and cereal, leafy vegetables, and dried fruits. Dried apricots and raisins are excellent iron-rich snacks for athletes. Have them wash the raisins and apricots down with orange juice because vitamin C is necessary in the intestinal tract for the absorption of iron.

30. ARE THERE ANY NUTRITIONAL PROBLEMS SPECI-FICALLY RELATED TO WOMEN? Yes, there are two other potential problems that should be discussed. One is menstruation. Normal menstruation involves a small loss of iron and protein, both of which will easily be replaced by good nutrition throughout the month. Approximately 5% of the female athletes will have excessive mentrual flows. These girls should be encouraged to increase their consumption of iron-rich foods, especially before and during their periods.

Another problem concerns the effects of birth control pills. Coaches and athletes should be aware that oral contraceptive pills may cause certain nutritional deficiencies in vitamin C, folic acid, and an essential amino acid, tryptophan. A well-balanced diet is especially important to women athletes taking these drugs.

CONCLUSION

Whatever you do, discourage the fad diets that athletes so often embrace! The characteristic inbalances of such diets can be particularly damaging during the important growing years. Remember, the key to "growing" and "going" is a variety of nutrients from the Basic Four Food Groups.

Acknowledgments

Portions of the following articles have been previously published by Ellington Darden in these magazines.

1. *Woman Coach* 1: 24, 25, 32, March-April 1975.

2. *Woman's World* 5: 20-23,February 1975.

3. *Pageant* 31: 29-33, December 1975.

6. *Scholastic Coach* 46: 54-56, September 1976.

8. *Athletic Journal* 56: 20,85-89, November 1975.

9. *Atlanta Sportsman* 1: 16, 17, 25, September 1975.

10. *Sky* 4: 38-40, December 1975; and *Air Line Pilot* 45: 22-25, March 1976.

11. *Strength and Health* 41: 40-41, 78, August 1973.

14. *Pageant* 31: 119-127, June 1976.

16. *Shape-Up* 1: 72-73, January 1974.

17. *Nutrition and Athletic Performance,* Pasadena, California: The Athletic Press, 1976.

18. *Journal of Home Economics* 64: 4-8, December 1972; and *Swimming World* 15: 44-45, February 1974.

20. *Clinical Medicine* 81: 21-23, July 1974.

23. *Strength and Health* 42: 50, 51, 65, April 1974; and *Strength and Health* 42: 56, 57, 64, 65, May 1974.

24. *Scholastic Coach* 46: 47-49, 71, December 1976.

About the Author

Ellington Darden, Ph.D., is Director of Research for Nautilus Sports/Medical Industries, DeLand, Florida. He is also Executive Program Director of the Athletic Center of Atlanta, Georgia.

Dr. Darden's educational background includes a B.S. in Recreation and a M.S. in Physical Education from Baylor University, and a Ph.D. in Physical Education from Florida State University. Also, he obtained two years of post-doctoral study in the Food and Nutrition Department at Florida State University.

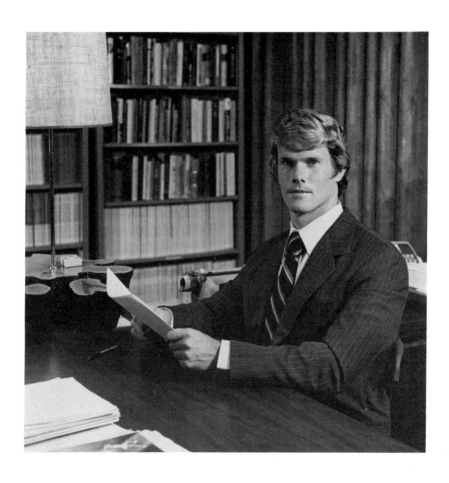